MY KIDNEY HEALTH

MY KIDNEY HEALTH

MANAGING POLYCYSTIC AND CHRONIC KIDNEY DISEASE

DR. JAMES KENNETH

Copyright

No part of this book should be copied, reproduced without the author's permission @2024 MY KIDNEY HEALTH BY DR. JAMES KENNETH

TABLE OF CONTENTS

Introduction --- 5
    Types of Kidney Disease ----------------------------------- 8
    Chronic kidney disease (CKD) ----------------------------- 8
PART 1 -- 10
Chronic kidney disease --- 10
    Diagnosis and screening ---------------------------------- 13
    1. Medical History and Physical Examination: ------ 14
    2. Laboratory Tests: -------------------------------------- 14
    3. Imaging Studies: --------------------------------------- 15
    4. Kidney Biopsy: --- 15
    5. Screening for High-Risk Populations: ------------ 16
Chapter 1 --- 17
The problem of kidney disease ------------------------------------ 17
    Signs and Symptoms ------------------------------------- 20
Four Ways to Prevent Kidney Disease Swelling --------- 25
    Preparing for your appointment ---------------------- 42
What you can do --- 42
What to expect from your doctor ---------------------------- 43
Chapter 2 --- 44
Stages Of CKD -- 44
Five stages of chronic kidney disease ---------------------- 44
Stage 1 kidney disease --- 45
Symptoms -- 45
Treatment --- 46
Stage 2 kidney disease --- 46
Symptoms -- 46
Treatment --- 47

Stage 3 kidney disease --------- 47
Symptoms --------- 48
Treatment --------- 48
Stage 4 kidney disease --------- 49
Symptoms --------- 50
Treatment --------- 51
Stage 5 kidney disease --------- 51
Symptoms --------- 52
Treatment --------- 52
Chapter 3 --------- 53
Complications and Causes --------- 53
Kidney failure --------- 53
Heart disease --------- 54
   Complications of chronic kidney disease --------- 55
Anemia --------- 55
Bone weakness --------- 56
Gout --------- 56
Heart disease --------- 57
Hyperkalemia --------- 57
Metabolic acidosis --------- 58
Uremia --------- 58
Weakened immune system --------- 58
Preventing complications --------- 59
Treating complications --------- 61
Chapter 4 --------- 62
How diet can help --------- 62
   Why is good nutrition important for people with kidney disease? --------- 63
   Other Nutrients --------- 68
   Foods to include for CKD --------- 76
   Foods to avoid in CKD --------- 83

Chapter 5 --87
Natural remedies and treatment ---------------------------87
   Is it safe to use herbal supplements if I have kidney
   disease? --87
   What are the facts about herbal supplements? -------88
   Which herbal supplements have potassium? ---------89
   Which herbal supplements have phosphorus? -------90
   Which herbal supplements should I avoid if I have
   kidney disease? ---91
   What about herbal supplements that act like a "water
   pill"? ---92
   Can herbal supplements interfere with the other
   medicines I take? --92
   Are there other health related issues for herbal
   supplements? --92
   What should I tell my doctor, dietitian or other
   healthcare provider? ---------------------------------------93
   The power of Baking Of Soda -------------------------93
   The great benefit of Activated Charcoal and Ginger
   Root ---99
   How does Turmeric affect CKD --------------------107
   Treatment for end-stage kidney disease-------------113
Dialysis--113
Kidney transplant --114
PART 2--115
Poly-cystic Kidney Disease --------------------------------115
Preparing for your appointment----------------------------117
Questions to ask your doctor ------------------------------118
What to expect from your doctor -------------------------119
Chapter 1--120
Unveiling Poly-cystic Disease -----------------------------120

Exercise and sports --------------------------------- 120
Signs and symptoms -------------------------------- 122
Chapter 2 -- 125
Managing symptoms and treatment approaches -------- 125
Treatment --- 129
Chapter 4 -- 131
Dietary supplement -------------------------------- 131
What to Eat --------------------------------------- 134
Chapter 4 -- 141
Natural remedies and complications ---------------- 141
Commonly used herbs in PDK ----------------------- 141
Complications ------------------------------------- 144
Chapter 5 -- 156
Caregiver and coping with PKD --------------------- 156
Additional Resources ------------------------------ 159

Introduction

Renal disease, also known as kidney disease, is a multifaceted medical condition that affects millions of individuals worldwide. The kidneys, two bean-shaped organs located on either side of the spine, play a vital role in filtering waste products and excess fluids from the bloodstream, regulating electrolyte balance, and producing hormones essential for various bodily functions. When the kidneys become damaged or dysfunctional, their ability to perform these critical tasks is compromised, leading to a wide range of health complications.

In this comprehensive guide, we will delve into the intricate world of renal disease, exploring its causes, symptoms, diagnosis, treatment options, and the profound impact it has on individuals, families, and communities. From the early stages of kidney damage to advanced renal failure, we will navigate the complexities of this condition, shedding light on the challenges faced by patients and caregivers alike.

One of the primary drivers of renal disease is chronic conditions such as diabetes and hypertension, which can gradually impair kidney function over time. Additionally, certain lifestyle factors, environmental toxins, genetic predispositions, and autoimmune disorders can contribute to the development and progression of kidney disease. Understanding these underlying causes is crucial for effective prevention and management strategies.

The symptoms of renal disease can vary widely depending on the stage and severity of the condition. Early signs may include fatigue, swelling of the extremities, changes in urine output, and elevated blood pressure. As the disease progresses, individuals may experience more pronounced symptoms such as persistent nausea, itching, muscle cramps, and difficulty breathing. Left untreated, renal disease can lead to serious complications, including cardiovascular disease, anemia, bone disorders, and ultimately, kidney failure.

Diagnosing renal disease typically involves a combination of medical history review, physical examination, laboratory tests, imaging studies, and kidney biopsy. Early detection is key to slowing the progression of the disease and preserving kidney function. Treatment options vary depending on the underlying cause and stage of renal disease but may include medications, lifestyle modifications, dialysis, and kidney transplantation.

Throughout this book, we will explore these topics in detail, providing insights from leading experts in the field, real-life patient experiences, and practical advice for navigating the complexities of renal disease. Whether you are a healthcare professional seeking to enhance your understanding of kidney health or an individual living with renal disease, this book aims to empower and educate, fostering a deeper appreciation for the importance of kidney health and wellness.

Types of Kidney Disease

Chronic kidney disease (CKD)

CKD is a condition where your kidneys can't filter toxins or extra fluid from your blood as well as they should. While the condition can vary in how serious it is, CKD usually gets worse over time. Treatment can slow the progression of the disease.

If left untreated, CKD may lead to kidney failure. At this stage, called end-stage renal disease (ESRD), the condition must be treated by dialysis or kidney transplant. Diabetes and high blood pressure are the leading causes of CKD.

It's estimated that 1 in 7 adult Americans have the condition. But 40% of those with serious chronic kidney disease aren't aware they have the condition.

Other common forms of kidney disease include:

Polycystic kidney disease: This genetic disorder causes cysts (fluid-filled sacs) to grow on your kidneys, limiting their ability to filter waste from your blood.

Lupus nephritis: Lupus is an autoimmune disease, meaning your immune system attacks healthy cells. Lupus nephritis is when your immune system attacks your kidneys.

Interstitial nephritis: This condition happens when you have a bad reaction to a medicine that limits your kidneys' ability to filter toxins. If you stop the medicine, your kidney health should improve.

PART 1

Chronic kidney disease

Chronic Kidney Disease (CKD) has a rich history intertwined with the evolution of medical knowledge and advancements in healthcare. The understanding of kidney function and the recognition of chronic kidney conditions have evolved over centuries.

The ancient Egyptians were among the first to recognize the importance of urine in diagnosing diseases, including kidney ailments. They observed changes in urine color, volume, and composition as indicators of health and disease. However, it wasn't until the 19th century that significant advancements were made in understanding kidney function and pathology.

In 1827, Richard Bright, an English physician, published a seminal work titled "Reports of Medical Cases," in which he described the clinical features and pathological findings of what is now known as Bright's disease, a term historically used to describe various kidney disorders. Bright's meticulous observations laid the foundation for the modern understanding of renal disease.

Throughout the 20th century, researchers made significant strides in unraveling the complexities of kidney function and dysfunction. Breakthroughs in nephrology, the branch of medicine dedicated to the study and treatment of kidney diseases, led to the development of diagnostic tests, treatment modalities, and renal replacement therapies such as dialysis and kidney transplantation.

In 2002, the National Kidney Foundation Kidney Disease Outcomes Quality Initiative (KDOQI) introduced a standardized definition and classification system for chronic kidney disease, marking a pivotal moment in the recognition and management of this condition. CKD was defined as the presence of kidney damage or decreased kidney function lasting for three months or more, irrespective of the underlying cause.

Today, chronic kidney disease represents a global public health challenge, with millions of people affected worldwide. It is associated with significant morbidity, mortality, and healthcare costs. Risk factors for CKD include diabetes, hypertension, obesity, smoking, and a family history of kidney disease.

Early detection and intervention are essential for slowing the progression of CKD and reducing the risk of complications. Screening tests such as blood pressure measurement, urine albumin-to-creatinine ratio, and estimated glomerular filtration rate (eGFR) play a crucial role in identifying individuals at risk and facilitating timely intervention.

As our understanding of kidney disease continues to evolve, ongoing research efforts aim to improve diagnostic techniques, develop targeted therapies, and enhance the quality of life for individuals living with chronic kidney disease. By raising awareness, promoting kidney health, and investing in research and education, we can work towards a future where kidney disease is better understood, preventable, and effectively managed

Diagnosis and screening

Diagnosing chronic kidney disease (CKD) requires a comprehensive approach that combines medical history review, physical examination, laboratory tests, imaging studies, and sometimes kidney biopsy. Early detection and accurate diagnosis are essential for initiating timely interventions to slow the progression of CKD and prevent complications. In this chapter, we will explore the various diagnostic methods and screening tools used to assess kidney function and detect CKD.

1. Medical History and Physical Examination:
   - A thorough medical history review and physical examination are the first steps in diagnosing CKD. Healthcare providers will inquire about symptoms, medical conditions, medications, family history, and lifestyle factors that may contribute to kidney disease. Physical examination may reveal signs such as edema, hypertension, and abnormalities in the abdomen or urinary system.

2. Laboratory Tests:

- Several laboratory tests are used to assess kidney function and detect abnormalities in blood and urine samples:
  - Serum Creatinine: Measurement of creatinine levels in the blood is used to estimate glomerular filtration rate (eGFR), a key indicator of kidney function. Elevated creatinine levels may suggest impaired kidney function.
  - Estimated Glomerular Filtration Rate (eGFR): Calculated based on serum creatinine levels, age, sex, and race, eGFR provides an estimate of kidney function and helps classify the stage of CKD.
  - Urinalysis: Analysis of urine samples for the presence of protein, blood, glucose, and other substances can indicate kidney damage or dysfunction.
  - Urine Albumin-to-Creatinine Ratio (ACR): ACR is used to assess urinary albumin excretion and detect early signs of kidney damage, especially in individuals with diabetes or hypertension.

3. Imaging Studies:
  - Imaging studies such as ultrasound, computed tomography (CT) scan, and magnetic resonance imaging (MRI) may be performed to visualize the structure and function of the kidneys and urinary tract. These tests can help identify structural

abnormalities, tumors, kidney stones, or obstructions that may contribute to CKD.

4. Kidney Biopsy:
   - In some cases, a kidney biopsy may be necessary to confirm the diagnosis of CKD and determine the underlying cause of kidney damage. During a biopsy, a small sample of kidney tissue is obtained and examined under a microscope to assess for signs of inflammation, scarring, or other abnormalities.

5. Screening for High-Risk Populations:
   - Certain populations, including individuals with diabetes, hypertension, cardiovascular disease, or a family history of kidney disease, are at higher risk for developing CKD. Screening programs targeting these high-risk groups may include regular monitoring of blood pressure, serum creatinine, and urinary albumin excretion to detect CKD at an early stage.

Early detection of CKD through routine screening and diagnostic testing allows for timely intervention and management strategies to slow the progression of the disease and reduce the risk of complications. Healthcare providers play a critical role in recognizing the signs and symptoms of CKD, conducting appropriate diagnostic evaluations, and implementing personalized treatment plans to optimize kidney health and overall well-being.

Chapter 1

The problem of kidney disease

Chronic kidney disease (CKD) represents a significant and growing public health challenge worldwide, affecting millions of individuals of all ages and backgrounds. This condition, characterized by the gradual loss of kidney function over time, poses numerous health risks and can lead to serious complications if left untreated.

One of the primary concerns surrounding CKD is its silent progression. In its early stages, CKD often presents with subtle or nonspecific symptoms, making it difficult to detect until significant kidney damage has occurred. This delayed diagnosis can delay intervention and exacerbate the progression of the disease, leading to more severe complications down the line.

Furthermore, CKD is closely linked with other chronic conditions such as diabetes, hypertension, and cardiovascular disease, forming a complex web of interconnected health issues known as the "chronic disease continuum." Individuals with these underlying conditions are at a higher risk of developing CKD, while CKD itself can further exacerbate the progression of these comorbidities, creating a vicious cycle of declining health.

Complications of CKD extend far beyond the kidneys themselves. As kidney function declines, the body's ability to regulate fluid balance, electrolytes, and waste products becomes compromised, leading to imbalances that can affect virtually every organ system. Cardiovascular complications, including hypertension, heart failure, and atherosclerosis, are particularly common among CKD patients and are a leading cause of morbidity and mortality.

Moreover, CKD significantly impacts quality of life for affected individuals. The burden of managing a chronic condition, undergoing regular medical treatments such as dialysis or transplantation, and coping with associated symptoms can take a toll on physical, emotional, and social wellbeing. Fatigue, depression, anxiety, and reduced mobility are just a few of the challenges faced by CKD patients on a daily basis.

The economic burden of CKD is also substantial, both for individuals and healthcare systems. The cost of medical care, including medications, dialysis treatments, hospitalizations, and transplant surgeries, can be prohibitively high, placing financial strain on patients and their families. Additionally, CKD-related productivity losses and disability further contribute to the socioeconomic impact of the disease.

Addressing the problem of chronic kidney disease requires a multifaceted approach that encompasses prevention, early detection, comprehensive management, and ongoing support for affected individuals. Public health initiatives aimed at raising awareness, promoting healthy lifestyles, and improving access to screening and treatment services are essential for reducing the burden of CKD on a global scale.

By recognizing the scale and complexity of the problem of chronic kidney disease and implementing effective strategies to address it, we can work towards a future where kidney health is prioritized, and individuals affected by CKD can live longer, healthier

Signs and Symptoms

Chronic kidney disease (CKD) is often referred to as a "silent disease" because it can progress slowly over time with few or no symptoms, especially in its early stages. However, as the condition advances, various signs and symptoms may become apparent, indicating declining kidney function and the need for medical evaluation and intervention. Understanding these signs and symptoms is crucial for early detection and management of CKD.

1. Fatigue and Weakness:
   - Feeling unusually tired, weak, or lacking in energy is a common symptom of CKD. As kidney function declines, toxins and waste products can build up in the bloodstream, leading to fatigue and lethargy.

1.Follow a Balanced Diet: Work with a dietitian to develop a meal plan that's tailored to your specific needs. A balanced diet that includes appropriate amounts of protein, carbohydrates, fats, vitamins, and minerals can help manage symptoms and maintain energy levels.

2. Manage Fluid Intake: Limiting fluids may be necessary if you're experiencing fluid retention or have been advised by your healthcare provider. However, dehydration can also cause fatigue, so it's essential to strike a balance. Consult with your healthcare team for personalized fluid intake recommendations.

3. Monitor Potassium and Phosphorus Levels: CKD can affect the body's ability to regulate potassium and phosphorus levels, which can contribute to weakness and fatigue. Be mindful of foods high in potassium and phosphorus, and follow your healthcare provider's recommendations for managing these levels.

4. Stay Active: Engage in regular physical activity, as tolerated. Exercise can help improve energy levels, strengthen muscles, and boost mood. Consult with your healthcare provider before starting any new exercise regimen to ensure it's safe for you.

5. Manage Anemia: Anemia is a common complication of CKD and can contribute to fatigue. Your healthcare provider may recommend iron supplements, erythropoiesis-stimulating agents

(ESAs), or other treatments to manage anemia and improve energy levels.

6. Get Adequate Rest: Prioritize quality sleep by maintaining a regular sleep schedule, creating a comfortable sleep environment, and practicing relaxation techniques before bedtime. Adequate rest is crucial for managing fatigue and promoting overall health.

7. Medication Management: Take medications as prescribed by your healthcare provider. Some medications may contribute to fatigue or interact with other medications, so it's essential to communicate any concerns or side effects with your healthcare team.

8. Manage Stress: Chronic stress can exacerbate fatigue and weaken the immune system. Practice stress-reduction techniques such as deep breathing, meditation, yoga, or hobbies that you enjoy to help manage stress levels.

9. Stay Hydrated: While fluid intake may be restricted, it's essential to stay adequately hydrated to prevent dehydration, which can worsen fatigue.

Follow your healthcare provider's guidance on fluid intake and monitor your hydration status regularly.

2. Changes in Urination:
The symptoms of changes in urine are very easy to see or smell. They typically include:

Changes in the color of your pee.
Strong odors coming from your pee.
Foaming or frothing of your pee.
Colors of pee

The color of your pee depends on how hydrated you are. If you drink a lot of fluid, your pee should be clear to yellow. If you're dehydrated, your pee is usually darker yellow or slightly orange. Other than how much fluid you drink, medication and foods can also affect the colors of your pee. But, pee that's red or dark brown may point to an underlying health condition.

Odor changes to pee

Your pee naturally has a smell that's unique to you. But, certain foods can alter the smell of your pee. If your pee takes on a sulfur smell, it may just mean you ate something like asparagus or you need to drink more water. Your pee should return to its normal smell within 24 hours or so. Strong-smelling or fishy-smelling pee that lasts longer than a day or two may be a sign that something else is going on.

Changes to the look of pee

Pee is typically clear. If your pee looks cloudy or foamy, it could indicate an infection or underlying medical condition. Like other urine changes, monitor how your pee looks to see if it's temporary. Peeing very quickly can make your pee foamy, as can eating certain foods. But if this issue persists — especially if you experience leg swelling — you should talk to your healthcare provider. It could be due to excess protein in your urine, a potential sign of kidney disease.

Four Ways to Prevent Kidney Disease Swelling

Making kidney-friendly lifestyle choices—such as eating well, taking the medications your doctor prescribes, and managing your fluid levels—may help you prevent swelling caused by kidney disease. Since your healthcare provider knows your medical history, they can tell you which lifestyle choices can benefit you the most and help you come up with a more detailed plan to avoid swelling. Ask them how the following tips can help you manage edema.

1. Avoid sodium

Sodium can cause fluid retention. Keeping it out of your diet can prevent excess fluid from building up in your body and also make you less thirsty. Avoid extra sodium by cooking your meals from scratch and shopping for fresh foods. Creating a grocery list before grocery shopping can also help you avoid foods with sodium.

2. Monitor blood pressure

High blood pressure may be an indication of excess fluid. Monitoring your blood pressure on a daily basis can help you stop edema before it happens. Talk to your care team about your ideal blood pressure and how to maintain it.

3. Weigh yourself daily

Gaining weight might mean your body has excess fluid, something you can monitor by weighing yourself daily. Get the most accurate number by doing this at the same time every day and wearing similar clothing. Record your weight each day so you can detect any change. Let your care team know if you do notice a rapid or drastic change—especially if you are also experiencing other symptoms like swelling or shortness of breath.

4. Decrease fluid intake

Decreasing your fluid intake can help you control your fluid levels. You can do this by eating frozen low-potassium fruits to quench your thirst. Try waiting 10 minutes for a fluid craving to pass. Lowering your sodium intake by choosing foods that have 10 percent or lower Daily Value of sodium which you can find on the Nutrition Facts label. Also, cooking with herbs and spices instead of salt can help reduce thirst and control fluid intake.

Learn ways to treat swelling

You can manage edema by following the treatments your doctor recommends. One of these treatments may be a prescription for a diuretic, also known as a water pill, which increases urine production and can help your kidneys remove the excess fluid in your body.

Dialysis is another treatment that can reduce swelling. If you're already on dialysis, complete each session, which can help remove excess fluid and reducing your swelling. If you go on dialysis in the future, make sure you know how long each session should be and how frequently you need it. Sticking to your full treatment is very important to remove all excess fluid. Also, talk to your care team about eating well on dialysis and other kidney-friendly lifestyle choices that can help minimize and sometimes avoid this uncomfortable symptom of kidney disease.

3. Swelling (Edema):
   - Edema, or swelling, commonly occurs in the legs, ankles, feet, and around the eyes in individuals with CKD. This swelling is due to the retention of fluids and electrolyte imbalances caused by impaired kidney function.

Swelling, also known as edema, is a common symptom in chronic kidney disease (CKD), especially in its advanced stages. It occurs when the kidneys are unable to remove excess fluid and waste from the body effectively, leading to fluid retention. Here are some tips for managing swelling associated with CKD:

1. Follow a Low-Sodium Diet: Sodium can contribute to fluid retention, so reducing your sodium intake can help decrease swelling. Avoid adding salt to your food, and limit your consumption of processed and packaged foods, which are often high in sodium.

2. Elevate Legs: Elevating your legs above heart level when sitting or lying down can help reduce swelling by encouraging fluid drainage from the legs back into the bloodstream.

3. Wear Compression Stockings: Compression stockings or socks can help prevent fluid buildup in the legs by applying gentle pressure to promote circulation. Consult with your health care provider to determine the appropriate type and fit for your needs.

4. Monitor Weight: Weigh yourself regularly and keep track of any significant changes in weight, as sudden weight gain can indicate fluid retention. Report any significant changes to your health care provider.

5. Take Medications as Prescribed: Your health-care provider may prescribe diuretics (water pills) to

help your kidneys remove excess fluid from your body. Take these medications exactly as prescribed and report any side effects or concerns to your healthcare provider.

6. Exercise Regularly: Gentle exercise, such as walking or swimming, can help improve circulation and reduce swelling. Consult with your health care provider before starting any new exercise regimen to ensure it's safe for you.

7. Manage Blood Pressure: High blood pressure can worsen swelling in CKD. Follow your health care provider's recommendations for managing blood pressure through lifestyle changes and medications, if necessary.

8. Avoid Prolonged Standing or Sitting: Limiting prolonged periods of standing or sitting can help prevent fluid from pooling in your legs and feet, which can worsen swelling. Take breaks to stretch and move around regularly.

4. Shortness of Breath:
   - Difficulty breathing or shortness of breath, especially during physical exertion, can occur as a

result of fluid buildup in the lungs (pulmonary edema) or anemia associated with CKD.

5. High Blood Pressure (Hypertension):

- Hypertension is both a cause and a consequence of CKD. High blood pressure can accelerate the progression of kidney damage, while CKD itself can lead to hypertension due to alterations in fluid and electrolyte balance and hormonal dysregulation.

Managing high blood pressure (hypertension) is crucial for individuals with chronic kidney disease (CKD), as it can further damage the kidneys and increase the risk of complications. Here are some tips for managing hypertension in CKD:

1.Follow a Healthy Diet: Adopt a diet rich in fruits, vegetables, whole grains, and lean proteins while limiting saturated fats, cholesterol, and sodium. The DASH (Dietary Approaches to Stop Hypertension) diet, which emphasizes fruits, vegetables, and low-fat dairy products, has been shown to help lower blood pressure.

2. Limit Sodium Intake: Reduce your sodium intake to help lower blood pressure and decrease fluid retention. Aim for no more than 2,300 milligrams of

sodium per day, or even lower if advised by your healthcare provider.

3. Maintain a Healthy Weight: Losing weight if you're overweight or obese can help lower blood pressure. Even modest weight loss can have a significant impact on blood pressure levels.

4. Limit Alcohol Consumption: Limit alcohol intake to no more than one drink per day for women and two drinks per day for men. Excessive alcohol consumption can raise blood pressure and contribute to kidney damage.

5. Quit Smoking: Smoking can raise blood pressure and accelerate kidney damage. If you smoke, talk to your healthcare provider about strategies to quit, such as counseling, nicotine replacement therapy, or prescription medications.

6. Take Medications as Prescribed: If lifestyle changes alone are not sufficient to control your blood pressure, your health care provider may prescribe medications such as ACE inhibitors, angiotensin II receptor blockers (ARBs), diuretics, or calcium channel blockers. Take these medications

exactly as prescribed and report any side effects to your health care provider.

7. Monitor Blood Pressure Regularly: Keep track of your blood pressure at home using a home blood pressure monitor, and report any significant changes to your health care provider. Consistently high blood pressure readings may require adjustments to your treatment plan.

6. Nausea and Vomiting:

- Persistent nausea, vomiting, and loss of appetite are common symptoms of advanced CKD. These symptoms may be related to uremia, a condition characterized by the buildup of waste products in the bloodstream.

Dealing with nausea can be uncomfortable, but there are several life hacks that may help alleviate the sensation:

1. Ginger: Ginger has natural anti-nausea properties. You can chew on a small piece of fresh ginger, drink ginger tea, or take ginger supplements to help calm your stomach.

2. Peppermint: Peppermint can help soothe nausea and calm the digestive system. Sip on peppermint tea or suck on peppermint candies to alleviate symptoms.

3. Acupressure: Applying pressure to specific points on the body, such as the wrist (known as the P6 or Nei Guan point), may help relieve nausea. You can use acupressure wristbands or simply apply pressure to the P6 point with your fingers.

4. Stay Hydrated: Sipping on clear fluids like water, herbal tea, or electrolyte-rich drinks can help prevent dehydration and ease nausea. Avoid drinking large amounts of fluid at once, as this can worsen nausea.

5. Eat Small, Frequent Meals: Instead of consuming large meals, opt for smaller, more frequent meals throughout the day. This can help prevent your stomach from becoming too full, which may trigger nausea.

6. Avoid Strong Odors: Strong smells can exacerbate feelings of nausea. Try to avoid strong-smelling foods, perfumes, or cleaning products, and opt for neutral or pleasant scents instead.

7. Rest and Relaxation: Stress and fatigue can worsen nausea. Practice relaxation techniques such as deep breathing, meditation, or gentle yoga to help calm your mind and body.

8. Cold Compress: Applying a cold compress or ice pack to the back of your neck or forehead may help alleviate nausea. The cold sensation can distract your brain from the feeling of nausea and provide relief.

7. Itching (Pruritus):
   - Pruritus, or severe itching, is a bothersome symptom experienced by many CKD patients. The exact cause of pruritus in CKD is not fully understood but may be related to the buildup of toxins, imbalances in calcium and phosphorus levels, or skin dryness.

These are excellent strategies for managing itching associated with chronic kidney disease. Here's a compiled list for easier reference:

1. Keep Your Skin Moisturized: Hydrate your skin regularly with fragrance-free moisturizers to prevent

dryness and itching. Apply moisturizer after bathing while your skin is still damp to lock in moisture.

2. Avoid Hot Water: Bathe or shower with lukewarm water instead of hot water, as hot water can strip your skin of its natural oils and exacerbate itching.

3. Use Gentle, Fragrance-Free Products: Opt for gentle, fragrance-free soaps, body washes, and laundry detergents to avoid further irritation to your skin. Harsh chemicals and fragrances can worsen itching.

4. Cool Compresses: Apply cool, damp cloths or ice packs to itchy areas to temporarily numb the skin and reduce inflammation. Avoid applying ice directly to the skin to prevent frostbite.

5. Wear Loose-Fitting Clothing: Choose loose-fitting, breathable clothing made from natural fabrics like cotton to minimize irritation and allow airflow to the skin. Tight clothing can exacerbate itching.

6. Avoid Scratching: Resisting the urge to scratch is crucial, as scratching can damage the skin and worsen itching. Instead, try gently patting or tapping

the itchy area to relieve the sensation without causing harm.

Incorporating these strategies into your daily routine can help manage itching associated with chronic kidney disease and improve your overall comfort and well-being. If itching persists or becomes severe, be sure to consult with your healthcare provider for further evaluation and treatment.

Herbal remedies
1. Aloe Vera: Aloe vera has soothing and moisturizing properties that can help relieve itching and reduce inflammation. Apply pure aloe vera gel directly to the itchy areas of the skin for relief.
2. Chamomile: Chamomile has anti-inflammatory and anti-itch properties. You can use chamomile tea bags to make a soothing compress or add chamomile essential oil to a carrier oil (such as coconut oil) and apply it topically to the skin.
3. Calendula: Calendula, also known as marigold, has anti-inflammatory and wound-healing properties. Calendula cream or ointment can be applied topically to soothe itching and promote healing.

4. Lavender: Lavender has calming and anti-inflammatory properties that can help alleviate itching and promote relaxation. Add a few drops of lavender essential oil to a carrier oil and apply it to the skin, or use lavender-scented products for a soothing effect.
5. Peppermint: Peppermint has cooling and numbing properties that can help relieve itching and reduce inflammation. You can use peppermint essential oil diluted in a carrier oil and apply it topically to the skin for relief.
6. Neem: Neem has antibacterial, antifungal, and anti-inflammatory properties that can help soothe itching and promote healing of the skin. Neem oil or neem cream can be applied topically to the affected areas.
7. Oatmeal: While not an herb, oatmeal has anti-inflammatory properties that can help relieve itching and soothe irritated skin. Add colloidal oatmeal to a warm bath or make a paste with oatmeal and water to apply to the skin.
8. Basil: Basil has anti-inflammatory and antimicrobial properties that can help alleviate itching and reduce irritation. Crush fresh basil leaves and apply the juice directly to the itchy areas of the skin for relief.

9. Licorice: Licorice root has anti-inflammatory properties that can help reduce itching and inflammation. You can apply licorice root extract topically to the skin or drink licorice tea for internal benefits.
10. Turmeric: Turmeric has anti-inflammatory and antioxidant properties that can help reduce itching and promote healing of the skin. You can apply a paste made from turmeric powder and water or mix turmeric powder into a carrier oil and apply it to the skin

8. Muscle Cramps and Restless Legs Syndrome (RLS):

- Muscle cramps, particularly in the legs, and restless legs syndrome (RLS), characterized by uncomfortable sensations in the legs and an irresistible urge to move them, are common complaints among individuals with CKD.

Muscle cramps and Restless Legs Syndrome (RLS) can be bothersome symptoms, especially for individuals with chronic kidney disease (CKD). Here are some tips to help manage these conditions:

1. Stay Hydrated: Dehydration can contribute to muscle cramps, so it's essential to stay adequately

hydrated. However, if you have CKD and are on fluid restrictions, be sure to follow your healthcare provider's recommendations for fluid intake.

2. Maintain Electrolyte Balance: Imbalances in electrolytes such as potassium, calcium, and magnesium can contribute to muscle cramps and RLS. Work with your healthcare provider to monitor and manage your electrolyte levels through diet and, if necessary, supplementation.

3. Stretching Exercises: Regular stretching exercises, particularly targeting the muscles prone to cramping, can help prevent and alleviate muscle cramps. Focus on stretching the calves, thighs, and feet.

4. Massage: Gentle massage of the affected muscles can help relax tight muscles and relieve muscle cramps. Use circular motions or apply pressure to the cramping muscle until the cramp subsides.

5. Heat and Cold Therapy: Applying heat or cold to the affected muscles can help alleviate muscle cramps and discomfort. Experiment with hot packs,

warm baths, cold packs, or ice massage to find what works best for you.

6. Avoid Triggers: Identify and avoid triggers that exacerbate RLS symptoms, such as caffeine, nicotine, alcohol, and certain medications. Additionally, avoid prolonged periods of sitting or standing, as this can worsen symptoms.

7. Establish a Sleep Routine: Stick to a regular sleep schedule and create a relaxing bedtime routine to help improve sleep quality and reduce RLS symptoms. Avoid stimulating activities close to bedtime, and create a comfortable sleep environment.

9. Cognitive Impairment:
   - CKD can affect cognitive function, leading to difficulties with concentration, memory, and mental processing speed. Cognitive impairment may result from the accumulation of uremic toxins, electrolyte imbalances, and cerebral microvascular disease.

10. Bone Pain and Fractures:
   - CKD can disrupt the balance of minerals in the body, leading to bone abnormalities and an

increased risk of fractures. Bone pain, particularly in the lower back and joints, may occur as a result of osteoporosis or renal osteodystrophy.

Recognizing these signs and symptoms of chronic kidney disease is essential for timely diagnosis and management. If you or someone you know is experiencing any of these symptoms, it is important to consult a healthcare professional for proper evaluation and treatment. Early intervention can help slow the progression of CKD and improve overall outcomes for affected individuals.

Preparing for your appointment

You'll likely start by seeing your primary care doctor. If lab tests reveal that you have kidney damage, you might be referred to a doctor who specializes in kidney problems (nephrologist).

What you can do

To get ready for your appointment, ask if there's anything you need to do ahead of time, such as limit your diet. Then make a list of:

- Your symptoms, including any that seem unrelated to your kidneys or urinary function, and when they began
- All your medications, vitamins or other supplements you take, including doses
- Other medical conditions you have and relatives with kidney disease
- Questions to ask about your condition

Take a family member or friend along, if possible, to help you remember the information you receive. Or use a recorder during your visit.

For chronic kidney disease, some basic questions to ask include:

- What's the level of damage to my kidneys?
- Is my kidney function worsening?
- Do I need more tests?
- What's causing my condition?
- Can the damage to my kidneys be reversed?
- What are my treatment options?
- What are the potential side effects of each treatment?
- I have these other health conditions. How can I best manage them together?
- Do I need to eat a special diet?

Can you refer me to a dietitian who can help me plan my meals?
Are there brochures or other printed material I can have? What websites do you recommend?
How often do I need to have my kidney function tested?
Don't hesitate to ask other questions as they occur to you.

What to expect from your doctor

Your doctor is likely to ask you questions, such as:

How long have you had symptoms?
Have you been diagnosed or treated for high blood pressure?
Have you noticed changes in your urinary habits?

Chapter 2

Stages Of CKD

With chronic kidney disease, the kidneys don't usually fail all at once. Instead, kidney disease often progresses slowly years. If caught early, medicines and lifestyle changes may help slow or prevent CKD progression.

Five stages of chronic kidney disease

The National Kidney Foundation (NKF) divided kidney disease into five stages. This helps doctors provide the best care, as each stage calls for different tests and treatments.

Doctors determine the stage of kidney disease using the glomerular filtration rate (GFR), a math formula using a person's age, gender, and their serum creatinine level (identified through a blood test). Creatinine, a waste product that comes from muscle activity, is a key indicator of kidney function. When kidneys are working well they remove creatinine from the blood; but as kidney function slows, blood levels of creatinine rise.

Stage 1 kidney disease

In stage 1, there's very mild damage to the kidneys. They're quite adaptable and can adjust for this, allowing them to keep performing at 90% or better.

At this stage, CKD is likely to be discovered by chance during routine blood and urine tests. You may also have these tests if you have diabetes or high blood pressure. These are the top causes of CKD in the United States, according to the National Institute of Diabetes and Digestive and Kidney Diseases (NIDDKD).

Symptoms
Typically, there are no symptoms when kidneys function at 90% or better.

Treatment
The NIDDKD suggests taking the following steps to help slow disease progression:

- Manage blood sugar levels if you have diabetes.
- Manage blood pressure if you have hypertension.
- Maintain a healthy, balanced diet.

- Don't use tobacco.
- Try to get 7–8 hours of sleep each night.
- Reduce stress and anxiety with relaxation techniques.
- Engage in physical activity for 30 minutes daily, at least 5 days a week.
- Try to maintain an appropriate weight for your body.
- A doctor may refer you to a kidney specialist, called a nephrologist. They can provide more tailored advice for you.

Stage 2 kidney disease

In stage 2 CKD, kidneys are functioning between 60–89%.

Symptoms
At this stage, you might still be symptom-free. Or symptoms are nonspecific, such as:

- Frequent urinary tract infections (UTIs)
- High blood pressure
- Swelling in your hands and feet
- Blood in your urine

Treatment

There's no cure for CKD, but following the NIDDKD's recommendations and early treatment can slow or stop progression.

It's essential to address the underlying cause and to manage any conditions, such as diabetes, high blood pressure, or heart disease.

Stage 3 kidney disease

Stage 3A CKD is when your kidney is functioning between 45–59%. Stage 3B means kidney function is between 30–44%.

The kidneys aren't filtering waste, toxins, and fluids well, which are starting to build up.

According to the NKF, this is the first stage when people are typically diagnosed with CKD because it's when an eGFR blood test alone can detect it.

Symptoms
Not everyone has symptoms at stage 3. However, you may experience:

- Back pain
- Fatigue

- Loss of appetite
- Persistent itching
- Sleep problems
- Swelling of the hands and feet
- Urinating more or less than usual
- Weakness

Complications may include:

- Anemia
- Bone disease
- High blood pressure

Treatment

A healthcare professional may recommend you make dietary changes, such as reducing your intake of sodium, calcium, potassium, and phosphorate. It's important to manage underlying conditions to help preserve kidney function. This may include taking:

- High blood pressure medications, such as angiotensin-converting enzyme (ACE) inhibitors or angiotensin II receptor blockers
- Diuretics to relieve fluid retention
- Cholesterol-lowering medications

- Erythropoietin supplements for anemia
- A healthcare professional may also recommend you stop taking some medications, such as nonsteroidal anti-inflammatory drugs (NSAIDs).

You may also require frequent follow-up visits and tests so adjustments can be made if necessary.

Stage 4 kidney disease

Stage 4 CKD means you have moderate-to-severe kidney damage. They're functioning between 15–29%, so you may build up more waste, toxins, and fluids in your body.

At this stage, it's important to do everything you can to prevent progression to kidney failure.

According to the Centers for Disease Control and Prevention (CDC), 40% of people with severely reduced kidney function aren't even aware they have it.

Symptoms
Symptoms can include:

- Back pain

- Chest pain
- Decreased mental sharpness
- Fatigue
- Loss of appetite
- Muscle twitches or cramps
- Nausea and vomiting
- Persistent itching
- Shortness of breath
- Sleep problems
- Swelling of the hands and feet
- Urinating more or less than usual
- Weakness
- Weight loss

Complications can include:

- Anemia
- Bone disease
- High blood pressure
- You're also at increased risk of heart disease and stroke.

Treatment
In stage 4, it's important to work closely with healthcare professionals. You should also start discussing treatments like dialysis and kidney transplants in case your kidneys fail.

In addition, stage 4 CKD can lead to further health complications requiring treatment. For example, it's not uncommon to develop metabolic acidosis due to CKD. Depending on blood bicarbonate levels, doctors may prescribe oral bicarbonate replacement therapy.

Stage 5 kidney disease

Stage 5 CKD means your kidneys are working at less than 15% capacity or you have kidney failure.

When this happens, the buildup of waste and toxins becomes life threatening. This is end-stage renal disease.

Symptoms
Symptoms of kidney failure can include:

- Back and chest pain
- Breathing problems
- Confusion and trouble focusing
- Weight losss
- Fatigue
- Little to no appetite
- Muscle twitches or cramps

- Nausea or vomiting
- Persistent itching
- Trouble sleeping
- Severe weakness
- Swelling of the hands and feet
- Urinating more or less than usual
- A significant drop in kidney function puts more stress on the heart, increasing the risk of heart disease and stroke.

Treatment

Once you have complete kidney failure, life expectancy is only a few months without dialysis or a kidney transplant.

Dialysis isn't a cure for CKD but a process to help remove waste and fluid from your blood. There are two types of dialysis: hemodialysis and peritoneal dialysis.

Chapter 3

Complications and Causes

Kidney failure
Kidney failure occurs when the kidneys are unable to filter waste effectively. When the kidneys filter less than 15% of waste from the blood, they cannot filter waste as quickly as your body produces it. This is known as end-stage kidney disease. It requires dialysis or a kidney transplant for survival.

Heart disease
Heart disease is a leading cause of death in people with kidney disease, particularly those on dialysis. Heart disease includes any disease that keeps your heart from pumping blood effectively.

Secondary hyperparathyroidism (SHPT)
You can develop hyperparathyroidism if your calcium levels get too low. It can cause symptoms that include:

- Joint swelling
- Fractures
- Bone disorders

- Neurological complications
- People with CKD have an increased risk of cerebrovascular disorders like stroke.

Those with end-stage kidney disease or on dialysis are more likely to have:

- Cognitive impairment
- Dementia
- Stroke, including ischemic, hemorrhagic, or silent strokes
- Poor long-term prognosis after a stroke
- Seizures
- Movement disorders, including Parkinson's disease

But neurological complications may occur in any stage of CKD.

Complications of chronic kidney disease

When your kidneys aren't working well, it can lead to complications in other areas of your body.

Potential concerns include:

Anemia

Being on dialysis can increase your risk of developing anemia. Anemia happens when your kidneys don't make enough erythropoietin (EPO). This affects their ability to make red blood cells. You may also have anemia due to low levels of: iron, vitamin B12, folic acid

Anemia can deprive vital organs and tissues of oxygen. If you have anemia, it can damage organs like your heart and brain. It can also worsen kidney function.

Bone weakness

CKD can lead to low calcium and high phosphorus levels (hyperphosphatemia), weakening your bones. This increases the risk of bone fractures.

You may also experience symptoms that include:

- Muscle spasms
- Mouth numbness and tingling
- Itchy skin
- Fluid retention

Fluid retention happens when your body hangs on to excess fluids. This can lead to: swelling of the limbs (edema), high blood pressure, fluid in the lungs

Gout

Gout is a type of arthritis caused by a buildup of uric acid in your joints. Uric acid is typically filtered out of your body through the kidneys. Doctors may recommend medications and dietary changes, including avoiding foods containing purines, which the body breaks down into uric acid. This can include: bacon, turkey, fish, dried beans, peas

Heart disease

When your kidneys aren't functioning well, they can't effectively filter waste from the blood. This leads to increased fluid in your blood, which may cause high blood pressure and heart damage.

High blood pressure (hypertension)
This happens when the force of the blood pumping through your blood vessels is too high.
Hypertension can lead to worsening kidney function,

which can cause fluid retention and worsening hypertension.

Hyperkalemia

If your kidneys cannot filter out excess potassium, it can build up in your blood. Hyperkalemia is a sudden rise in potassium levels that may affect heart function.

If you have kidney disease, you may need to limit foods high in potassium.

Metabolic acidosis

When there's too much acid in your bodily fluids that your kidneys don't filter out, it disturbs the pH balance of your blood. This can worsen kidney disease and lead to issues like bone or muscle loss and endocrine disorders.

Uremia

Uremia is a buildup of waste products in your blood. It is an indicator of severe kidney damage and often occurs in the later stages of kidney failure. It can cause a variety of symptoms, such as fatigue, nausea, restless legs, sleep disturbances

Weakened immune system

If you have chronic kidney disease, you may be more susceptible to infection and illness. People who are immunocompromised may need to take certain precautions to avoid illnesses. These can include:
- Following vaccination recommendations
- Avoid potential exposures to illness
- Take food safety precautions
- Oral care

Secondary complications

Depression is a common disorder among people with chronic conditions like CKD.
Depression may be due to psychosocial and biological changes that go along with dialysis. Depression in CKD is associated with: poor quality of life, adverse medical outcomes, increased mortality

Other secondary complications can include:
skin infections from dry skin and scratching

joint, bone, and muscle pain, nerve damage, a buildup of fluid around the lungs (pleural effusion), liver failure, sleep disorders

Preventing complications

At any stage of CKD, working closely with a doctor is important.

There's no cure for CKD. But you can slow its progression and lower your chances of developing related health complications.

Getting routine blood work and urinalyses will help catch health issues early on. A doctor typically monitors your kidney function by keeping an eye on your estimated glomerular filtration rate (eGFR) and urine albumin.

A healthcare team can also help you manage health concerns like diabetes, cholesterol, and weight.

Other things you can do to help prevent complications include

- Talk with a dietitian to make sure you're meeting your nutritional needs.

- Get regular physical activity.
- Reach and maintain a moderate weight.
- Get 7 to 8 hours of sleep each night.
- Avoid smoking and exposure to second-hand smoke, or quit smoking, if you smoke.
- Learn coping mechanisms to deal with stress, anxiety, or depression. A doctor can refer you to a mental health professional or support group for help.
- Take prescribed medications as directed.
- Be cautious with over-the-counter (OTC) medications. Nonsteroidal anti-inflammatory drugs (NSAIDs) can harm your kidneys. Check with a doctor or pharmacist before taking new OTC medications.

Treating complications

Treating CKD complications can help improve related symptoms and overall quality of life. Left untreated, certain complications of CKD may become life threatening.

Anemia
Treating anemia may help reduce the risk of additional complications. Treatment can include:

erythropoiesis-stimulating agents, which tell your body to produce more red blood cells
iron supplements
blood transfusions
High blood pressure

If you have high blood pressure, treatment may include:
Eating a nutritious diet
Regular physical activity, such as walking,
Swimming, and yoga
Medications to lower blood pressure

Other complications

Other treatments depend on specific symptoms and what's causing them.

If you progress to end-stage kidney failure, you'll likely need dialysis or a kidney transplant.

Chapter 4

How diet can help

Nutrition is all about eating a healthy and balanced diet so your body gets the nutrients that it needs. Nutrients are substances in foods that our bodies need to function and grow.

Why is good nutrition important for people with kidney disease?

Making healthy food choices is the key to better mental and physical health and it is even more important if you have chronic kidney disease (CKD).

Eating nutritious foods gives you more energy and can help you:
- Do your daily tasks
- Prevent infection
- Build muscle
- Help maintain a healthy weight

- Manage your kidney disease and keep it from getting worse Will I need to change my diet? There is no single eating plan that is right for eve

Will I need to change my diet?

There is no single eating plan that is right for everyone with kidney disease. The best foods for you depends on how well your kidneys works and other factors, like if you have diabetes. Your doctor can refer you to a kidney dietitian (a dietitian who specializes in kidney disease) who can teach you how to choose foods that are right for you.

How can a kidney dietitian help?

A kidney dietitian can:
- Help you choose foods that will give you the right nutrients in the right amounts
- Explain why diet changes are important
- Answer your questions

Nutrition basics
A healthy eating plan gives you the right amount of:
- Protein
- Calories
- Vitamins

- Minerals

Healthy diet plans for people with kidney disease

- Mediterranean diet
(CKD stages 1–5 not on dialysis)
- Diets high in fruits and vegetables
(CKD stages 1–4)
- Other options include DASH and plant-based diets

Why do I need protein?

Protein is an important nutrient. Your body needs protein to help build muscle, repair tissue, and fight infection. But if you have kidney disease, you may need to closely watch the amount of protein you eat to prevent protein wastes from building up in your blood. This can help your kidneys work longer. Your doctor will tell you if you need to limit how much protein you eat each day. Decisions are based on your stage of kidney disease, level of nutrition, muscle mass, and other things. Let your kidney doctor and kidney dietitian help you.

Protein comes from the following:

- Lentils and dried beans
- Unsalted nuts
- Fish and other seafood
- Eggs
- Poultry (chicken and turkey
- Meats (beef, veal, lamb, pork).

Your kidney dietitian can help you learn how to maintain good nutrition and eat the right amount of protein to help your kidneys and prevent muscle breakdown.

How many calories do I need?

Every person is different. Calories are like fuel—they provide your body with the energy you need to live. They are important because they:
- Help you stay at a healthy body weight
- Give you energy to do your daily tasks and remain active
- Help your body use the protein in food to build muscles and tissues

It is important to plan meals that give you enough

calories each day. Otherwise, your body may not have energy to stay healthy. Your kidney dietitian can help you do this. Some people may be told to eat more calories. They may need to eat extra sweets like sugar, jam, jelly, hard candy, honey, and syrup. Other good sources of calories come from fats such as unsalted nuts and oils like canola or olive oil.

How do I get enough vitamins and minerals?

Most people get enough vitamins and minerals to stay healthy by eating a wide variety of foods each day. However, if you have kidney disease, you may need to limit some foods that would normally give you these important vitamins and minerals. If so, you may need to take special vitamins or minerals instead. Your doctor and kidney dietitian will tell you what choice are good for you.

How will I know if I am getting enough calories and nutrients?

Your doctor will test your blood and urine. These tests will help show whether or not you are getting enough nutrients. Your kidney dietitian may also ask you about the foods you eat. You may also be asked to keep track of everything you eat or drink, also known as a "food diary."

What if I don't want to eat or don't like my food choices?

When you have kidney disease, it may be difficult to get enough nutrients from food, especially if you are on a limited-protein diet. Many people with kidney disease also find it hard to eat enough calories each day.
Many supplements are available, and some are made just for people with kidney disease or diabetes. Check with your doctor or kidney dietitian before taking any supplements.

Will I need nutritional supplements?

Remember, not all people with kidney disease have the same dietary needs. Your doctor and kidney dietitian will tell you if you need to take nutritional supplements. Use only the supplements recommended by your doctor or kidney dietitian.

Other Nutrients

Will I need to control any other nutrients?
You may need to balance fluids and other important nutrients. They are:
- Sodium
- Phosphorus
- Calcium
- Potassium

SODIUM

Sodium is a mineral found in most foods. It is also found in table salt. Sodium affects blood pressure and water balance in your body.

Healthy kidneys can control sodium. But, if your kidneys do not work well, sodium and fluid build up in your body. This can cause high blood pressure and other problems, like swelling of your ankles, fingers, or eyes. Your doctor or kidney dietitian will tell you if you need to limit sodium.

You can limit sodium by limiting table salt and foods such as:
- Seasonings like soy sauce, sea salt, teriyaki sauce, garlic salt, onion salt, or seasoned salt
- Most canned foods and frozen dinners (unless they say "low sodium" check the label)

- Processed meats like ham, bacon, hot dogs, sausage, and deli meats
- Salted snack foods, like chips and crackers
- Canned or dehydrated soups (like packaged noodle soup)
- Most restaurant foods, takeout foods, and fast foods.

Your kidney dietitian can teach you how to choose lower sodium foods. Learning how to read food labels can help you find foods with less sodium.

PHOSPHORUS

Phosphorus is a mineral found in many foods. People with kidney disease may need to closely watch how much phosphorus is in their food. As kidney disease gets worse, the kidneys are not able to remove extra phosphorus. Large amounts of phosphorus are found in:

- Dairy products such as milk, cheese, yogurt, ice cream, and pudding
- Nuts and peanut butter
- Nondairy creamer
- Beverages such as cocoa, beer, and dark cola drinks
- Pancake mix
- Processed, convenience, and fast foods,

including meats that have phosphate additives to make them tender

Eating high-phosphorus foods can raise the level of phosphorus in your blood. However, phosphorus from plant foods is less absorbed than phosphorus from animal foods or phosphate additives.

What happens when phosphorus builds up in your blood?

Your blood calcium levels drop and calcium is pulled from the bones. Over time, your bones will become weak and break easily. A high level of phosphorus in your blood may also cause calcium to build up in your blood vessels, heart, joints, muscles,and skin, where it does not belong. This may cause serious problems such as:
- Damage to the heart and other organs
- Poor blood circulation
- Bone pain
- Skin ulcers

To keep phosphorus at safe levels in your blood, you may need to limit phosphorus-rich foods. You may also need to take a type of medicine called a phosphate binder. These binders are taken with your meals and snacks to block some of the phosphorus from the foods you eat from entering your body.

Your doctor and kidney dietitian will tell you if you need to limit high-phosphorus foods or take phosphate binders.

CALCIUM

Calcium is a mineral that is important for building strong bones. However, foods that are good sources of calcium are often high in phosphorus. The best way to prevent calcium loss from your bones is to limit high-phosphorus foods.

You may also need to take phosphate binders and avoid eating calcium-fortified foods. Your doctor may also recommend that you take a special form of vitamin D to help keep calcium and phosphorus levels in balance, and to prevent bone disease.

POTASSIUM

Potassium is another important mineral found in most foods. Potassium helps your muscles and heart work properly. Large amounts of potassium are found in:

• Certain fruits and vegetables (like bananas, melons, oranges, potatoes, tomatoes, dried fruits, nuts, avocados, dark colored and leafy green vegetables, and some juices)

- Milk and yogurt
- Dried beans and peas
- Potassium chloride salt substitutes
- Protein-rich foods, such as meat, poultry, pork, and fish.

A simple blood test can check your potassium level. Too much or too little potassium in the blood can be dangerous. Some people with kidney disease need more potassium; others need less. How much you need depends on how well your kidneys are working.

It also depends on whether or not you are taking any medicine that changes the level of potassium in your blood.

FLUID

Most people in the early stages of with kidney disease do not need to limit the amount of fluids they drink. If you do not know your stage of kidney disease, ask your doctor.

If your kidney disease gets worse, your doctor will let you know if you need to limit fluids and how much fluid is okay for you each day. To avoid dehydration, let your doctor and kidney dietitian help plan your fluid intake.

What if I have diabetes?

You may need to make a few changes in your diet if you have diabetes and kidney disease. If your doctor says that you should eat less protein, your diet may need to include more carbohydrates or high-quality fats to give you enough calories. Work with your kidney dietitian to make a meal plan that is right for you.

Ask your doctor how often to test your blood sugar levels. Try to keep your levels under control. Your dosage of insulin or other medicines may need to change if your kidney disease gets worse. Contact your doctor if your blood sugar levels are too high or too low.

What about plant-based or meatless diets?

Plant-based or meatless diets may have a positive effect on health. Eating a variety of plant foods and getting enough calories is important. Without enough calories, your body will break down the protein you eat to create energy instead. If protein is broken down, more waste products have to be removed by your kidneys.

Ask about ways to check that the amount of protein you are eating is right for you. Talk with your kidney dietitian about the best sources of plant protein that have the right amounts of potassium and phosphorus to best meet your dietary needs. Your doctor or kidney dietitian can check your blood to make sure you are getting the right amount of protein and calories.

How is nutritional health is checked?

You will be checked regularly by your doctor and dietitian to make sure you are getting the right nutrients that you need. Some tests are:

PHYSICAL NUTRITION EXAM

Your dietitian may give you an exam to check your body for signs of nutrition problems. This exam is called a Subjective Global Assessment (SGA). Your dietitian asks you about the foods you eat and looks at the fat and muscle levels in your body.
The dietitian notes:
• Changes in your weight
• Changes in the tissues around your face, arms, hands, shoulders, and legs
• Your food intake
• Your activity and energy levels
• Problems that might interfere with eating

DIETARY INTERVIEWS AND FOOD DIARIES

Your dietitian will ask about what you eat. You may also be asked to keep a food diary of everything you eat and drink each day. Your dietitian wants to see if you are getting the right amount protein, calories, vitamines and minerals.

Questions for your healthcare professional

If you have questions or are unsure about anything, write down your questions before you go to your doctor or kidney dietitian because it is easy to forget what you wanted to talk about.
Make sure you ask what each test result means and what your options are. You need to understand the treatment plan that your doctor or dietitian thinks is good for you. This is your health, so never feel uncomfortable about asking anything.

Foods to include for CKD

Chronic Kidney Disease (CKD) necessitates careful dietary management to support kidney function and overall health. The right foods can help mitigate symptoms, manage complications, and slow the progression of CKD. Here's a detailed guide on foods to include for individuals with CKD and the reasons behind their inclusion:

1. Low-Potassium Fruits and Vegetables: Opt for fruits and vegetables with lower potassium content to prevent hyperkalemia, a condition characterized by high levels of potassium in the blood. Suitable choices include apples, berries, grapes, green beans, and cabbage.

2. Low-Phosphorus Foods: Phosphorus buildup is common in CKD and can lead to bone and heart problems. Incorporate foods low in phosphorus such as white bread, rice, cauliflower, and cucumbers.

3. Lean Proteins: High-quality protein sources are vital for maintaining muscle mass without overloading the kidneys. Include lean meats like chicken and turkey, fish (preferably low-mercury options like salmon and trout), and plant-based proteins such as tofu and legumes.

4. Limited Sodium: Excessive sodium can contribute to fluid retention and high blood pressure,

worsening CKD symptoms. Opt for fresh or homemade meals seasoned with herbs and spices instead of salt. Avoid processed foods, canned soups, and fast food, which are typically high in sodium.

5. Healthy Fats: Incorporate unsaturated fats like those found in olive oil, avocados, and nuts. These fats support heart health and provide essential nutrients without adding extra stress to the kidneys.

6. Moderate Portions of Whole Grains: Whole grains like brown rice, quinoa, and whole wheat bread provide fiber and essential nutrients while helping to manage blood sugar levels. However, portion control is crucial as they contain some phosphorus and potassium.

7. Limited Dairy Products: Dairy products are high in phosphorus and potassium, so consume them in moderation. Opt for low-phosphorus alternatives like almond milk or small servings of low-fat dairy products if tolerated.

8. Controlled Fluid Intake: Fluid restriction may be necessary, especially in later stages of CKD. Monitor fluid intake, including water, soups, and

other beverages, based on individual recommendations from healthcare providers.

9. Herbs and Spices: Flavor meals with herbs and spices like garlic, ginger, basil, and cinnamon to enhance taste without adding extra sodium or potassium.

10. Supervised Vitamin and Mineral Supplements: CKD can lead to deficiencies in vitamins and minerals such as vitamin D, calcium, and iron. Work with a healthcare provider to determine appropriate supplements to meet individual needs.

The reasons behind including these foods in a CKD-friendly diet are multifaceted:

- Nutrient Balance: By focusing on low-potassium and low-phosphorus options, individuals can maintain a better balance of essential nutrients, reducing the strain on compromised kidneys.

- Blood Pressure Management: Limiting sodium intake helps manage blood pressure, reducing the risk of complications such as cardiovascular disease and further kidney damage.

- Protein Quality: Opting for lean proteins supports muscle health without overloading the kidneys with excess waste products from protein metabolism.

- Fluid Control: Monitoring fluid intake is crucial for individuals with CKD to prevent fluid overload, which can lead to edema, hypertension, and other complications.

- Overall Health Maintenance: A well-rounded CKD diet promotes overall health, including heart health, bone health, and blood sugar management, which are all important considerations for individuals with kidney disease.

In conclusion, a CKD-friendly diet emphasizes nutrient balance, portion control, and mindful food choices to support kidney function and overall well-being. By incorporating the suggested foods and following individualized dietary recommendations, individuals with CKD can better manage their condition and improve their quality of life.

Breakfast, lunch and dinner ideas

Breakfast:

1. Oatmeal made with water, topped with sliced strawberries and a sprinkle of chopped almonds.
2. Smoothie made with almond milk, spinach, banana, and a scoop of protein powder.
3. Whole grain cereal with low-fat milk or almond milk, topped with sliced peaches.
4. Egg white omelette with diced bell peppers, onions, and tomatoes, served with a slice of whole grain toast.
5. Cottage cheese mixed with diced pineapple or peaches, served with a small portion of whole grain crackers.

Lunch:

1. Turkey and avocado wrap made with a whole grain tortilla, lettuce, and tomato.
2. Lentil soup with carrots, celery, and kale, served with a side salad of mixed greens and balsamic vinaigrette.
3. Tuna salad made with canned tuna in water, mixed with Greek yogurt, diced cucumbers, and cherry tomatoes, served on whole grain bread.
4. Grilled vegetable and quinoa salad with a lemon-tahini dressing.

5. Black bean and corn salsa with baked tortilla chips, served with a side of sliced bell peppers and hummus.

Dinner:

1. Grilled chicken breast with roasted sweet potatoes and steamed broccoli.
2. Stir-fried tofu with bell peppers, snap peas, and carrots, served over brown rice.
3. Baked cod with a side of sautéed spinach and quinoa pilaf.
4. Vegetable curry made with chickpeas, cauliflower, and spinach, served with a side of basmati rice.
5. Turkey chili made with lean ground turkey, kidney beans, diced tomatoes, and spices, served with a side of cornbread made with cornmeal.

Snacks:

1. Rice cake topped with almond butter and banana slices.
2. Celery sticks filled with cream cheese and topped with dried cranberries.
3. Greek yogurt with a drizzle of honey and a sprinkle of sunflower seeds.

4. Apple slices dipped in unsweetened almond butter.
5. Air-popped popcorn sprinkled with nutritional yeast and black pepper.

These meal ideas offer a variety of flavors and textures while adhering to CKD dietary guidelines. Remember to monitor portion sizes and adjust recipes as needed based on individual nutritional requirements and restrictions.

Foods to avoid in CKD

1. High-Potassium Foods
   - Bananas: A medium-sized banana contains about 400 mg of potassium.
   - Oranges and orange juice: A cup of orange juice contains approximately 450 mg of potassium.
   - Potatoes (especially sweet potatoes): A medium-sized baked potato contains around 900 mg of potassium.
   - Tomatoes and tomato products: A cup of tomato sauce can contain up to 900 mg of potassium.

2. High-Phosphorus Foods

- Dairy products: Milk, cheese, and yogurt are high in phosphorus. For example, one cup of milk contains around 250 mg of phosphorus.
- Nuts and seeds: Almonds, peanuts, and sunflower seeds are rich in phosphorus. A quarter cup of almonds contains approximately 140 mg of phosphorus.
- Whole grains: Whole wheat bread, brown rice, and whole grain pasta are high in phosphorus. For instance, one slice of whole wheat bread contains about 60 mg of phosphorus.

3. High-Sodium Foods

- Processed and packaged foods: Items like canned soups, frozen meals, and snack foods are often high in sodium. For example, one serving of canned soup can contain over 800 mg of sodium.
- Deli meats and cured meats: Bacon, ham, and salami are examples of high-sodium meats. Two slices of bacon can contain around 300 mg of sodium.
- Condiments and sauces: Soy sauce, barbecue sauce, and salad dressings can be high in sodium. Just one tablespoon of soy sauce contains approximately 1,000 mg of sodium.

4. Processed and Fast Foods

- Fast food burgers and fries: A typical fast food cheeseburger and small fries can contain over 1,000 calories and high amounts of sodium and unhealthy fats.
- Frozen pizza: Frozen pizzas often contain high levels of sodium, saturated fat, and processed meats.
- Packaged snacks: Chips, crackers, and cookies are examples of processed snacks that are high in sodium, unhealthy fats, and sometimes phosphorus additives.

5. High-Protein Foods

- Red meat: Beef, pork, and lamb are high in protein and should be consumed in moderation. For example, a 3-ounce serving of beef steak contains about 25 grams of protein.
- Processed meats: Sausages, hot dogs, and bacon are examples of processed meats high in protein and sodium.
- High-fat dairy products: Full-fat cheese and ice cream are high in protein and should be limited due to their saturated fat content.

6. High-Purine Foods

- Organ meats: Liver and kidney are high in purines and should be avoided. For instance, a 3-

ounce serving of beef liver contains approximately 370 mg of purines.

- Certain seafood: Anchovies, sardines, and mussels are high in purines. A 3-ounce serving of anchovies contains around 500 mg of purines.

- Meat extracts: Bouillon cubes and meat extracts like beef or chicken broth are high in purines and should be used sparingly.

7. High-Sugar Foods

- Sugary beverages: Soda, energy drinks, and sweetened fruit juices can contain high amounts of added sugars. For example, a 12-ounce can of cola contains around 39 grams of sugar.

- Candy and sweets: Candies, chocolates, and pastries are high in sugar and should be limited in a CKD diet.

- Sweetened cereals: Many breakfast cereals are high in sugar, with some containing over 10 grams of sugar per serving.

8. Alcohol

- Beer, wine, and spirits: Alcoholic beverages should be limited or avoided due to their potential negative effects on kidney function and interactions with medications.

Avoiding these foods can help individuals with CKD better manage their condition, control symptoms, and improve overall health outcomes. It's important to work with a healthcare provider or dietitian to develop a personalized nutrition plan tailored to individual needs and stage of kidney disease.

Chapter 5

Natural remedies and treatment

Is it safe to use herbal supplements if I have kidney disease?

You may think about using herbal supplements to help with any health concerns you may have, but as a patient with kidney disease, you should use caution with herbal supplements.
Use of herbal supplements is often unsafe if you have kidney disease since some herbal products can cause harm to your kidneys and even make your kidney disease worse. Also, your kidneys cannot clear waste products that can build up in your body.
The herbal supplement market is a multi-million dollar business. You may hear from a friend or family member about an herbal supplement that they think has improved their health or well-being and they suggest it to you. While this advice may be fine for them, it can be dangerous for you with kidney disease.

What are the facts about herbal supplements?

The following facts about herbal supplements are true for everyone, with or without kidney disease. Herbal supplements often have more than one name: a common name and a plant name. Some common concerns include:

The Food and Drug Administration (FDA) does not regulate herbal supplements for dose, content, or pureness.

Some herbal supplements have aristolochic acid, which is harmful to kidneys.

Herbal supplements made in other countries may have heavy metals.

There are few studies to show if herbal supplements have real benefits and even less information in patients with kidney disease.

Herbal supplements may interact with prescription medicines to either decrease or increase how the medicine works.

Which herbal supplements have potassium?

Potassium is a mineral that may need to be limited in the diet of people with kidney disease especially for those on dialysis. Herbal supplements that have potassium include:

Alfalfa	American Ginseng	Bai Zhi (root)
Bitter Melon (fruit, leaf)	Black Mustard (leaf)	Blessed Thistle
Chervit (leaf)	Chicory (leaf)	Chinese Boxthorn (leaf)
Coriander (leaf)	Dandelion (root, leaf)	Dulse
Evening Primrose	Feverfew	Garlic (leaf)
Genipap (fruit)	Goto Kola	Japanese Honeysuckle (flower)
Kelp	Kudzu (shoot)	Lemongrass
Mugwort	Noni	Papaya (leaf, fruit)
Purslane Sage (leaf)	Safflower (flower)	Sassafras
Scullcap	Shepherd's Purse	Stinging Nettle (leaf)
Turmeric (rhizome)	Water Lotus	

Which herbal supplements have phosphorus?

Phosphorus is a mineral that may need to be limited in the diet of people with kidney disease especially for those on dialysis. Some herbal supplements that have phosphorus include:

American Ginseng	Bitter Melon	Borage (leaf)
Buchu (leaf)	Coriander (leaf)	Evening Primrose
Feverfew	Flaxseed (seed)	Horseradish (root)
Indian Sorrel (seed)	Milk Thistle	Onion (leaf)
Pokeweed (shoot)	Purslane	Shepherd's Purse
Silk Cotton Tree (seed)	Stinging Nettle (leaf)	Sunflower (seed)
Turmeric (rhizome)	Water Lotus	Yellow Dock

Which herbal supplements should I avoid if I have kidney disease?

Herbal supplements that are especially risky for patients with any stage of kidney disease, who are on dialysis or who have a kidney transplant include:

Astragalus	Barberry	Cat's Claw
Apium Graveolens	Creatine	Goldenrod
Horsetail	Huperzinea	Java Tea Leaf
Licorice Root	Nettle, Stinging Nettle	Oregon Grape Root
Parsley Root	Pennyroyal	Ruta Graveolens
Uva Ursi	Yohimbe	

What about herbal supplements that act like a "water pill"?

Some herbal supplements that act like a diuretic or "water pill" may cause "kidney irritation" or damage. These include bucha leaves and juniper berries. Uva Ursi and parsley capsules may also have bad side effects.

Can herbal supplements interfere with the other medicines I take?

Many herbal supplements can interact with prescription drugs. A few examples are St. Johns Wort, echinacea, ginkgo, garlic, ginseng, ginger, and blue cohosh. If you have a kidney transplant you are especially at risk, as any interaction between herbal supplements and medicines could put you at risk for losing your kidney.

Are there other health related issues for herbal supplements?

As with anyone, patients with kidney disease may have other health related issues. If you have a history of a bleeding disorder you are at high risk for bad reactions to herbal supplements. Women who are pregnant or lactating, as well as children, are also at high risk.

What should I tell my doctor, dietitian or other healthcare provider?

In general, it is not recommended for patients with kidney disease to use herbal supplements. If you choose to take one, always tell your doctor, dietitian, or other health care provider. Always update the use of herbal supplements at your visits to your healthcare provider as a medication change.

The power of Baking Of Soda

The benefits of treating metabolic acidosis with sodium bicarbonate include:

- Preventing more severe metabolic acidosis
- Slowing CKD progression
- Preventing complications of CKD progression, such as:
    - Bone loss
    - Muscle loss
    - Malnutrition
    - Insulin resistance
    - Cardiovascular complications
- Improving nutritional status

Based on current evidence, the Kidney Disease Improving Global Outcomes Guidelines for CKD suggest sodium bicarbonate is successful at increasing serum bicarbonate levels and preventing more severe acidosis and potential complications.

Are there side effects of treating kidney disease with sodium bicarbonate?

When ingested, sodium bicarbonate produces carbon dioxide (CO_2) gas, which can lead to common gastrointestinal side effects, such as bloating and belching.

Other side effects may include:

- Unpleasant taste
- Headache
- Nausea or vomiting
- Increased need to urinate
- Nervousness or restlessness

In very rare cases, consuming sodium bicarbonate can cause a rupture of the stomach due to increased intragastric pressure from several factors, including CO_2 with food and liquid in the stomach.

For this reason, only take sodium bicarbonate on an empty stomach, and don't take the total daily dose at one time.

What are the risks of treatment treating kidney disease with sodium bicarbonate?

One potential risk of sodium bicarbonate treatment is an increased intake of sodium.

Sodium bicarbonate is a chemical compound that combines sodium (salt) and bicarbonate, so daily treatment with sodium bicarbonate can lead to a substantial increase in sodium intake.

In people with CKD, increased sodium may contribute to:

- weight gain
- fluid retention
- swelling (edema)
- hypertension

High sodium intake also may prevent certain CKD treatments, such as rein-angiotensin-aldosterone system inhibitors, from working as well to slow the progression of kidney disease.

Other potential risks of sodium bicarbonate treatment include exceeding regular serum bicarbonate levels, which can lead to health difficulties, and vascular and kidney calcification.

With careful monitoring from a healthcare professional, sodium bicarbonate treatment is generally safe and well-tolerated.

What's the outlook for people with kidney disease who take sodium bicarbonate?

The outlook for people with CKD receiving treatment with sodium bicarbonate depends on the severity and stage of CKD as well as the severity of metabolic acidosis.

Without treatment, metabolic acidosis can lead to serious complications including CKD progression, osteoporosis, muscle loss, and death.

Effective treatments for metabolic acidosis include dietary changes, such as eating more alkali-containing fruits and vegetables, and medications such as sodium bicarbonate. These treatments may help improve your outlook if you have kidney disease.

How to use Baking Soda in CDK

Baking soda, or sodium bicarbonate, has been suggested as a potential adjunct therapy for chronic kidney disease (CKD), particularly in the context of managing metabolic acidosis, a common complication of advanced CKD. However, its use should be approached cautiously and under the guidance of a healthcare professional, as improper dosage or use can lead to adverse effects, including metabolic alkalosis, electrolyte imbalances, and worsening kidney function. Here are some considerations for using baking soda in CKD:

1. Evaluation of acid-base balance: Baking soda is primarily used to counteract metabolic acidosis, a condition characterized by an imbalance in the body's acid-base levels, often seen in advanced CKD. Your healthcare provider may perform blood tests to assess your acid-base status and determine if baking soda therapy is appropriate for you.

2. Dosage and administration: If your healthcare provider determines that baking soda therapy is suitable for managing metabolic acidosis, they will prescribe the appropriate dosage and administration schedule. Baking soda is typically taken orally in the form of tablets or powder dissolved in water. It's essential to follow your healthcare provider's instructions carefully to avoid complications.

3. Monitoring and follow-up: Regular monitoring of kidney function, electrolyte levels, and acid-base status is essential when using baking soda therapy in CKD. Your healthcare provider will schedule follow-up appointments to assess your response to treatment, make any necessary adjustments to

dosage or medication regimen, and address any concerns or side effects.

4. Adherence to dietary restrictions: In addition to baking soda therapy, managing CKD often involves dietary modifications to control electrolyte levels, fluid intake, and protein consumption. It's essential to adhere to any dietary restrictions recommended by your healthcare provider to optimize kidney function and overall health.

5. Potential side effects and precautions: While baking soda therapy can be beneficial in managing metabolic acidosis, it's not without risks. Common side effects include gastrointestinal discomfort, bloating, and gas. Long-term use of baking soda may also exacerbate hypertension and worsen kidney function in some individuals. Therefore, it's crucial to discuss potential risks and benefits with your healthcare provider before initiating therapy.

In summary, baking soda may have a role in managing metabolic acidosis in CKD, but its use should be carefully monitored and guided by a healthcare professional. Open communication with your healthcare provider is essential to ensure safe and effective treatment and to address any concerns or complications that may arise.

The great benefit of Activated Charcoal and Ginger Root

Activated charcoal and ginger root are often discussed for their potential health benefits, but their specific advantages and risks in the context of chronic kidney disease (CKD) warrant careful consideration. Here's a more detailed exploration:

Activated Charcoal

Recognized for its ability to adsorb toxins and chemicals, activated charcoal is proposed to have potential benefits for individuals with CKD. Given that CKD can compromise the kidneys' ability to effectively filter waste products, activated charcoal might theoretically aid by binding to toxins in the gastrointestinal tract, preventing their absorption into the bloodstream. However, robust clinical evidence supporting its efficacy in CKD is lacking. Moreover, activated charcoal has the potential to interfere with the absorption of medications and essential nutrients. This is particularly critical for

CKD patients who often have complex medication regimens and specific dietary requirements. Therefore, the utilization of activated charcoal in CKD should be approached cautiously and under the guidance of a healthcare professional.

How to use Activated Charcoal

Activated charcoal is a highly absorbent substance that has various uses, including as a remedy for certain gastrointestinal issues, detoxification, and poisoning emergencies. However, its use should be approached with caution, and it's essential to consult with a healthcare professional before using it, especially if you have any underlying health conditions or are taking medications. Here are some general guidelines for using activated charcoal:

1. Consultation with a healthcare provider: Before using activated charcoal, it's crucial to consult with a healthcare provider to determine if it's appropriate for your specific situation. They can provide guidance on dosage, administration, and potential risks or interactions with medications.

2. Administration: Activated charcoal is typically available in powder, capsule, or suspension form.

It's usually taken orally, either mixed with water or in capsule form with plenty of water. Follow the dosage instructions provided by your healthcare provider or the product label carefully.

3. Timing: Activated charcoal is most effective when taken on an empty stomach, away from meals and medications. It's important to space out the timing of activated charcoal consumption from other medications or supplements to prevent interference with their absorption.

4. Dosage: The recommended dosage of activated charcoal can vary depending on the reason for use and individual factors such as age, weight, and health status. Your healthcare provider will determine the appropriate dosage for you based on these factors. Avoid exceeding the recommended dosage unless instructed by a healthcare professional.

5. Hydration: It's essential to drink plenty of water when taking activated charcoal to prevent dehydration, especially if you're experiencing diarrhea or vomiting. Adequate hydration helps prevent constipation and ensures the proper passage of charcoal through the digestive tract.

6. Monitoring and follow-up: After taking activated charcoal, monitor your symptoms and response to treatment. If you experience any adverse reactions or if your symptoms persist or worsen, seek medical attention promptly. Follow up with your healthcare provider as recommended for further evaluation and management.

7. Precautions: Activated charcoal can interfere with the absorption of medications and nutrients in the digestive tract. Therefore, it's essential to avoid taking activated charcoal close to the time of taking medications or essential nutrients. Your healthcare provider can advise you on the appropriate timing to minimize potential interactions.

8. Storage: Store activated charcoal products according to the manufacturer's instructions, typically in a cool, dry place away from moisture and heat. Follow any specific storage recommendations provided on the product label.

Remember that activated charcoal is not a substitute for medical treatment, and its use should be part of a comprehensive treatment plan under the guidance of a healthcare professional. If you have any questions or concerns about using activated charcoal, don't hesitate to discuss them with your healthcare provider.

Ginger Root

It has a long history of use for its anti-inflammatory and digestive properties. In the context of CKD, ginger holds potential benefits such as reducing inflammation and alleviating symptoms like nausea and vomiting, which are prevalent in CKD patients undergoing dialysis or experiencing uremia. However, it's important to note that ginger contains oxalates, compounds that can contribute to kidney stone formation. As such, moderation is key when incorporating ginger into the diet or considering ginger supplements for individuals with CKD. Consulting with a healthcare provider is essential to determine appropriate usage, especially considering individual health status and potential interactions with medications.

It's crucial to approach dietary supplements and alternative treatments with caution. Open communication with healthcare providers is vital to ensure that any interventions, including the incorporation of activated charcoal or ginger root, are safe and aligned with overall treatment goals. Emphasizing a balanced diet tailored to individual needs remains fundamental in managing CKD effectively, alongside regular monitoring and adjustment of treatment plans as needed.

How to use Ginger Root

Ginger root is a versatile ingredient known for its distinct flavor and potential health benefits, including anti-inflammatory and digestive properties. Here's how you can use ginger root in various forms:

1. Fresh ginger root:
   - Peel the ginger root using a vegetable peeler or the edge of a spoon to remove the skin.
   - Slice, chop, or grate the ginger according to your recipe or preference.
   - Add fresh ginger to soups, stews, stir-fries, marinades, sauces, salads, and smoothies for a flavorful kick.
   - Brew ginger tea by steeping fresh ginger slices in hot water for several minutes. You can add lemon, honey, or other herbs for additional flavor.

2. Dried ginger powder:
   - Dried ginger powder is a convenient option for adding ginger flavor to dishes.

- Use it as a spice in cooking and baking, such as in curry blends, spice rubs, cookies, cakes, and bread.
- Mix dried ginger powder with hot water or tea to make a quick ginger infusion.

3. Ginger supplements:
- Ginger supplements, including capsules, extracts, and tinctures, are available for those who prefer a concentrated form of ginger.
- Follow the dosage instructions provided on the supplement packaging or as recommended by a healthcare professional.

4. Ginger essential oil:
- Ginger essential oil is potent and should be used with caution. It can be added to massage oils, diffusers, or baths for aromatherapy purposes.
- When using ginger essential oil topically, always dilute it with a carrier oil to avoid skin irritation.

Tips for using ginger root effectively and safely:

- Start with a small amount of ginger and adjust according to taste preferences.

- Store fresh ginger root in the refrigerator or freezer to prolong its shelf life. It can also be stored at room temperature in a cool, dry place.
- When purchasing ginger supplements or essential oil, choose reputable brands and consult with a healthcare professional, especially if you have any underlying health conditions or are pregnant or breastfeeding.
- If you experience any adverse reactions after consuming ginger or using ginger products, discontinue use and consult a healthcare professional.
- Ginger can interact with certain medications, so it's essential to discuss its use with your healthcare provider if you're taking medications or have any health concerns.

Incorporating ginger root into your diet can add both flavor and potential health benefits. Experiment with different forms and recipes to find enjoyable ways to include ginger in your meals and beverages.

How does Turmeric affect CKD

Turmeric has long been used in traditional eastern medicine for its health benefits. Curcumin, which is the main bioactive component in turmeric, is a powerful antioxidant with anti-inflammatory properties.

However, while turmeric and curcumin are generally safe to consume, too much of a good thing can be dangerous. One of the risks is that large doses can be bad for your kidneys. That's because too much curcumin can significantly increase the levels of urinary oxalate in your body, increasing the risk of kidney stone formation.

What are the negative effects of turmeric?

There are other potential risks to taking too much curcumin, including:
Mild side effects include upset stomach, acid reflux, diarrhea, dizziness and headaches.
Since turmeric acts as a blood thinner, it should be avoided if you have a bleeding disorder.
Turmeric can interact negatively with medications including blood thinners, antidepressants, antibiotics, antihistamines, cardiac medications and chemotherapy treatments. It can also interfere with diabetes medications and result in dangerously low blood sugar levels.

Turmeric can aggravate stomach problems, such as acid reflux and gallstones.

Since turmeric limits iron absorption, you shouldn't take it if you are on iron supplements.

Women who are pregnant or breastfeeding can eat food that contains turmeric as a spice but should avoid taking turmeric supplements. These supplements may stimulate uterus contractions and cause complications.

Depending on your overall health and whether you have conditions like gastrointestinal disorders or kidney stones, you should speak with your doctor before taking turmeric supplements.

How much turmeric is safe to consume?

Studies that show the health benefits of turmeric use turmeric extracts that contain mostly curcumin in doses exceeding 1 gram per day. Since it's difficult to consume that much naturally in a regular diet, turmeric is often taken as a supplement, where the curcumin content is much higher.

Generally speaking, an acceptable amount of curcumin supplement to take on a daily basis is about 1.4 milligrams per pound of body weight, up to 12 grams. Anything more than that can cause you to have adverse reactions.

What are the potential health benefits of turmeric?

Numerous preclinical trials have shown promising effects of curcumin in the treatment of heart disease, arthritis, Alzheimer's disease, gastrointestinal disorders and metabolic syndrome.

When consumed in moderation, turmeric can have significant health benefits:

- Anti-inflammatory properties: Curcumin has strong anti-inflammatory properties and can be as effective as anti-inflammatory medications but without the side effects. It can help to reduce chronic inflammation in joints and wounds, alleviating swelling, pain and discomfort. Because inflammation is often at the root of certain chronic diseases, turmeric can be used to treat conditions like rheumatoid arthritis, inflammatory bowel disease and pancreatitis.

- Pain relief: Curcumin can reduce rheumatoid arthritis pain, as well as gastrointestinal pain associated with inflammatory bowel disease.

- Antioxidant properties: Turmeric has strong antioxidant properties and protects the body from the free radicals that damage healthy cells. It can combat aging and boost metabolism, as well as reduce the risk of heart disease, cancer, cataracts, glaucoma and macular degeneration (age-related eye changes).

- Immunity booster: Turmeric's natural antiseptic, antibacterial, antiviral and antifungal properties help stimulate the immune system and protect the body from infection.

- Reduces cancer risk: Research has shown that turmeric can destroy cancerous cells, interfering with the growth, development and spread of cancer at a molecular level. Turmeric may especially play a vital role in treating and preventing cancers of the digestive system, such as colorectal cancer. It can also help counteract the effects of carcinogenic additives in processed food.

- Lowers heart disease risk: The antioxidant and anti-inflammatory properties of curcumin may prevent heart diseases and cardiovascular complications. Curcumin also reduces low-density lipoproteins (LDL), or bad cholesterol, preventing atherosclerosis.

- Diabetes prevention: Curcumin delays the onset of type 2 diabetes. Turmeric supplements taken along with metformin may help people with type 2 diabetes stabilize their blood sugar levels.

- Alzheimer's disease prevention: Curcumin clears the buildup of protein tangles in the brain called amyloid plaques, which are linked to Alzheimer's disease.

- Reduces depression: Curcumin boosts levels of neurotrophic factors in the brain, as well as neurotransmitters, serotonin and dopamine, all of which can help people with symptoms of depression.

- Aids digestion: Turmeric stimulates the gallbladder to produce bile, making the digestive system more efficient. Turmeric also aids enzymatic reactions, acid production and optimal

absorption of nutrients in the gut and can reduce bloating.
- Liver detox: Turmeric can increase the production of vital enzymes that help in breaking down and removing toxins in the liver. Turmeric also promotes good liver health by improving blood circulation.

- Improves bone health: Curcumin supplements can help improve joint function, prevent bone loss and preserve bone tissue.

- Promotes good skin: Because of its anti-inflammatory, antimicrobial and antioxidant properties, turmeric may help to:

◆ Lighten dark circles
◆ Prevent acne
◆ Give a natural glow
◆ Heal wounds
◆ Reduce scars
◆ Reduce eczema and psoriasis
◆ Delay wrinkles

Turmeric does not absorb into the body easily when taken alone. So in order to achieve maximum health benefits, turmeric should be consumed with black pepper, which contains a compound called piperine that boosts the absorption of turmeric in the body.

Treatment for end-stage kidney disease

If your kidneys can't keep up with waste and fluid clearance on their own and you develop complete or near-complete kidney failure, you have end-stage kidney disease. At that point, you need dialysis or a kidney transplant.

Dialysis

Dialysis artificially removes waste products and extra fluid from your blood when your kidneys can no longer do this. In hemodialysis, a machine filters waste and excess fluids from your blood.

In peritoneal dialysis, a thin tube inserted into your abdomen fills your abdominal cavity with a dialysis solution that absorbs waste and excess fluids. After a time, the dialysis solution drains from your body, carrying the waste with it.

Kidney transplant

A kidney transplant involves surgically placing a healthy kidney from a donor into your body. Transplanted kidneys can come from deceased or living donors.

After a transplant, you'll need to take medications for the rest of your life to keep your body from rejecting the new organ. You don't need to be on dialysis to have a kidney transplant.

For some who choose not to have dialysis or a kidney transplant, a third option is to treat your kidney failure with conservative measures. Conservative measures likely will include symptom management, advance care planning and care to keep you comfortable (palliative care).

PART 2

Poly-cystic Kidney Disease

Poly-cystic kidney disease (PKD) is a hereditary condition characterized by the growth of fluid-filled cysts in the kidneys, leading to kidney enlargement and eventual loss of function. With a prevalence of approximately 1 in 500 individuals worldwide, PKD represents a significant health concern affecting people of all ages and ethnicity. In this brief overview, we will explore the history and fundamentals of PKD, shedding light on its historical context, causes, symptoms, and the impact it has on individuals and families.

The history of poly-cystic kidney disease dates back centuries, with early descriptions of the condition found in ancient medical texts. However, it wasn't until the 20th century that significant advancements were made in understanding PKD as a distinct clinical entity.

In 1856, the French physician Rayer provided one of the earliest clinical descriptions of PKD, referring to it as "interstitial nephritis with cysts." Over the following decades, researchers made incremental progress in elucidating the pathology and genetic basis of the disease.

In the 20th century, the advent of modern genetics and molecular biology revolutionized our understanding of PKD. In 1963, Potter proposed a classification system for PKD based on cystic morphology and inheritance patterns. Subsequent studies identified mutations in specific genes associated with PKD, including PKD1 and PKD2, which encode proteins involved in renal tubule development and function.

The identification of these genetic mutations paved the way for diagnostic testing and genetic counseling for individuals at risk of inheriting PKD. Moreover, advances in imaging technology, such as ultrasound, computed tomography (CT), and magnetic resonance imaging (MRI), enabled clinicians to visualize cystic changes in the kidneys with greater precision and accuracy.

Today, ongoing research efforts continue to unravel the complexities of PKD, with a focus on developing targeted therapies to slow disease progression and improve outcomes for affected individuals. Despite the challenges posed by PKD, advancements in genetics, imaging, and therapeutic interventions offer hope for the future, underscoring the importance of continued research and collaboration in the fight against this debilitating condition.

When to see a doctor
It's not uncommon for people to have poly-cystic kidney disease for years without knowing it.

If you develop some of the signs and symptoms of poly-cystic kidney disease, see your doctor. If you have a first-degree relative — parent, sibling or child — with poly-cystic kidney disease, see your doctor to discuss screening for this disorder.

Preparing for your appointment

You're likely to start by seeing your primary care provider. However, you might be referred to a doctor who specializes in kidney health (nephrologist). You may benefit from starting a specialized treatment early on in the course of the disease, even if blood tests show that you still have normal kidney function.

Here's some information to help you get ready for your appointment.

What you can do?

When you make the appointment, ask if there's anything you need to do in advance, such as fasting before having a specific test. Make a list of:

Your symptoms, including any that seem unrelated to the reason for which you scheduled the appointment, and when they began
All medications, vitamins and other supplements you take, including dosages
Your and your family's medical history, particularly kidney diseases

Questions to ask your doctor

Take a family member or friend along, if possible, to help you remember the information you receive.

For polycystic kidney disease, questions to ask your doctor include:

- What's the most likely cause of my symptoms?
- Are there other possible causes for my symptoms?
- What tests do I need?
- Is this condition temporary or chronic?
- What's the best course of action?
- What alternatives are there to the approach you're suggesting?
- I have other health conditions. How can I best manage them together?
- Do I need to restrict my diet or activities?
- Are there brochures or other printed material that I can take?
- What websites do you recommend?

Don't hesitate to ask other questions.

What to expect from your doctor

Your doctor is likely to ask you questions, such as:
- Have your symptoms been continuous or occasional?
- Does anything seem to improve or worsen your symptoms?
- Do you know what your blood pressure normally is?
- Has your kidney function been measured?

Chapter 1

Unveiling Poly-cystic Disease

Poly-cystic kidney disease (PKD) can have a significant impact on an individual's lifestyle due to the physical, emotional, and practical challenges associated with the condition.

Exercise and sports

Exercise is an important part of maintaining good, overall health. Regular exercise can decrease your blood pressure and stress as well as improve muscle strength, heart function and stamina. It can also enhance a sense of well-being. In general, you will do much better on dialysis and with a transplant if you are physically fit.

What kind of exercise is best?

There is no one best kind of exercise. The key is to find an activity that is comfortable for you and that you enjoy doing. Generally, PKD patients can do any activity they want unless they get blood in the urine or it causes back, flank or abdominal pain. The exercises that are least jarring to the kidneys include walking, swimming and biking.

Be sure to talk with your doctor before starting an exercise regimen, as he or she may have guidance about what will be most effective for you, or what to avoid. Remember to always keep well hydrated when exercising, and do your best to be active on a regular basis.

Are sports dangerous to my kidneys?

In general, most sports do not affect kidney function. However, PKD does present unique circumstances and so there are some issues that need to be considered. Given the unique nature of PKD, where kidneys are enlarged and cysts can rupture, there are some simple precautions to take. Contact sports where the kidneys may be traumatized (flank/side or lower back impact) should either be avoided or protective pads should be worn. Examples of these types of sports include football, rugby, basketball, hockey and particularly boxing or kickboxing. Horseback riding and cross-country biking are other sports with repetitive impact that could potentially cause issues with your kidneys. There is no evidence that these activities worsen renal function, but they can result in pain and/or blood appearing in the urine.

Diet and nutrition

There are many reasons to maintain a healthy diet as a PKD patient including the potential to slow cyst growth, diabetes, and faster transplant recovery times.

Signs and symptoms

Signs and symptoms of polycystic kidney disease (PKD) can vary widely among individuals and may change over time as the condition progresses. While some individuals may experience mild symptoms or remain asymptomatic for years, others may develop more severe symptoms and complications. Here are common signs and symptoms associated with PKD:

1. Abdominal or Flank Pain:

Pain in the abdomen or flank region is one of the most common symptoms of PKD. The pain may be dull, intermittent, or sharp and may be caused by the enlargement of the kidneys or the presence of cysts pressing on surrounding tissues.

2. Hematuria:
Hematuria, or blood in the urine, can occur in individuals with PKD due to the presence of cysts in the kidneys that can rupture or bleed. Hematuria may present as pink, red, or cola-colored urine and may be accompanied by other urinary symptoms such as urgency or frequency.

3. Hypertension (High Blood Pressure):
High blood pressure is a common complication of PKD and may develop early in the course of the disease. Hypertension can accelerate the progression of kidney damage and increase the risk of cardiovascular complications such as heart disease and stroke.

4. Enlarged Kidneys:
As cysts accumulate in the kidneys, they can cause the kidneys to become enlarged, leading to abdominal distension or palpable masses in the abdomen. Enlarged kidneys may be detected during

a physical examination or imaging studies such as ultrasound, CT scan, or MRI.

5. Urinary Tract Infections (UTIs):

Individuals with PKD may be at increased risk of urinary tract infections due to cysts obstructing urinary flow and creating a favorable environment for bacterial growth. Symptoms of UTIs may include pain or burning with urination, increased urinary frequency, urgency, and cloudy or foul-smelling urine.

6. Kidney Stones:

Kidney stones are another common complication of PKD and can cause severe pain, urinary symptoms, and complications such as obstruction and infection. Individuals with PKD may have a higher risk of developing kidney stones due to altered kidney anatomy and function.

7. Proteinuria:

Proteinuria, or the presence of protein in the urine, may occur in individuals with PKD as a result of kidney damage. Proteinuria may be detected through urine tests and may indicate impaired kidney function and increased risk of progression to kidney failure.

Chapter 2

Managing symptoms and treatment approaches

The severity of poly-cystic kidney disease varies from person to person — even among members of the same family. Often, people with PKD reach end-stage kidney disease between ages 55 to 65. But some people with PKD have a mild disease and might never progress to end-stage kidney disease.

Treating poly-cystic kidney disease involves dealing with the following signs, symptoms and complications in their early stages:

- Kidney cyst growth: Tolvaptan therapy may be recommended for adults at risk of rapidly progressive ADPKD. Tolvaptan (Jynarque, Samsca) is a pill that you take by mouth that works to slow the rate of kidney cyst growth and the decline in how well your kidneys work.

- There's a risk of serious liver injury when taking tolvaptan, and it can interact with other medicines you take. It's best to see a doctor who specializes in kidney health (nephrologist) when taking tolvaptan, so that you can be monitored for side effects and possible complications.

- High blood pressure: Controlling high blood pressure can delay the progression of the disease and slow further kidney damage. Combining a low-sodium, low-fat diet that's moderate in protein and calorie content with not smoking, increasing exercise and reducing stress may help control high blood pressure.

- However, medications are usually needed to control high blood pressure. Medications called angiotensin-converting enzyme (ACE) inhibitors or angiotensin II receptor blockers (ARBs) are often used to control high blood pressure.

- Declining kidney function: To help your kidneys stay as healthy as possible for as long as possible, experts recommend maintaining a normal body weight (body mass index). Drinking water and fluids throughout the day may help slow the growth of kidney cysts, which in turn could slow down a decline in kidney function. Following a low-salt diet and eating less protein might allow kidney cysts to respond better to the increase in fluids.

- Pain: You might be able to control the pain of poly-cystic kidney disease with over-the-counter medications containing acetaminophen. For some people, however, the pain is more severe and constant. Your doctor might recommend a procedure using a needle to draw out cyst fluid and inject a medication (sclerosing agent) to shrink kidney cysts. Or you may need surgery to remove cysts if they're large enough to cause pressure and pain.

- Bladder or kidney infections: Prompt treatment of infections with antibiotics is necessary to prevent kidney damage. Your doctor may investigate whether you have a simple bladder infection or a more complicated cyst or kidney infection. For more complicated infections, you may need to take a longer course of antibiotics.

- Blood in the urine: You'll need to drink lots of fluids, preferably plain water, as soon as you notice blood in your urine to dilute the urine. Dilution might help prevent obstructive clots from forming in your urinary tract. In most cases, the bleeding will stop on its own. If it doesn't, it's important to contact your doctor.

- Kidney failure: If your kidneys lose their ability to remove waste products and extra fluids from your blood, you'll eventually need either dialysis or a kidney transplant. Seeing your doctor regularly for monitoring of PKD allows for the best timing of a kidney transplant. You may be able to have a preemptive kidney transplant, which means you wouldn't need to start dialysis but would have the transplant instead.

- Aneurysms: If you have poly-cystic kidney disease and a family history of ruptured brain (intracranial) aneurysms, your doctor may recommend regular screening for intracranial aneurysms.

If an aneurysm is discovered, surgical clipping of the aneurysm to reduce the risk of bleeding may be an option, depending on its size. Nonsurgical treatment of small aneurysms may involve controlling high blood pressure and high blood cholesterol, as well as quitting smoking.

Is poly-cystic kidney disease preventable?

Poly-cystic kidney disease isn't preventable. But you may be able to slow the disease or prevent kidney failure by practicing a healthy lifestyle.

Treatment

What is the treatment for polycystic kidney disease?

The most common treatments for PKD include:
- Blood pressure management: Your provider helps you manage your blood pressure with medicine, diet and exercise. Keeping your blood pressure within a safe range reduces your risk of heart disease and stroke.

- Breathing support: Infants with underdeveloped lungs and breathing problems may need mechanical ventilation.
- Dialysis: If you have kidney failure, you may need dialysis (a procedure to clean the blood). Hemodialysis uses a machine to filter blood outside the body. Peritoneal dialysis uses the lining of your belly and a special fluid to filter blood.
- Growth therapy: Underweight or underdeveloped infants may need help growing. A healthcare provider may recommend nutritional therapy or human growth hormone.
- Kidney transplant: You may need a kidney transplant if ADPKD progresses to end-stage renal failure. A transplant is surgery to replace a failing kidney with a donor kidney.
- Pain management: Medicine can manage pain caused by infections, kidney stones or burst cysts. Your healthcare provider should approve any pain medicines you take. Some medicines can make kidney damage worse.

Chapter 4

Dietary supplement

Although autosomal dominant poly-cystic kidney disease (ADPKD) does not have a cure, diet appears to have some influence on the condition by protecting the kidneys of individuals who have ADPKD.

By working closely with your kidney specialist and a nutrition expert, kidney-protective diets may help individuals with ADPKD slow the progression of poly-cystic kidney disease and damage to the kidneys.

Benefits

ADPKD is a progressive disease that, over time, will affect kidney function and cause permanent damage. Dietary modifications with this chronic kidney disease are important to preserve kidney function for as long as possible.

One study specific to individuals affected by ADPKD showed success with a small number of participants in preparing and following a diet specifically designed for ADPKD. Many other studies have shown the correlation between dietary modifications and stabilizing kidney function as well.

In diseases like ADPKD in which kidney function is impaired, the kidneys are not able to filter fluid as well, which results in the body keeping more sodium, or salt, than needed. Increased sodium has been studied extensively. It directly affects blood pressure, often raising it so consistently that individuals with ADPKD also have a diagnosis of hypertension, or high blood pressure.

When dietary salt intake is decreased, the body maintains a better sodium balance and keeps blood pressure within acceptable ranges. This same effect occurs with potassium and phosphorus. So, following a diet containing foods lower in potassium and phosphorus can help the body maintain a proper balance and prevent a more rapid decline to total kidney failure.

Another dietary recommendation includes limiting animal protein. Doing so has been shown to restrict growth of the cysts and minimize deterioration of overall kidney function. How animal protein causes cyst growth is unknown, but there is enough research indicating a diet high in animal protein causes more cysts and hastens progression to full kidney failure.

Drinking water, with the goal to balance water intake against kidney function to prevent fluid excess, helps the kidneys to maintain fluid balance more effectively. Minimizing dark sodas and caffeine is also important to maintain the fluid balance that allows the kidneys to work as optimally as possible.

How It Works

Following a recommended diet specific to chronic kidney disease like ADPKD is important to preserving kidney function and delaying kidney function decline.

Duration

Since ADPKD is a progressive disease with no known cure, developing a diet appropriate for maintaining kidney function for as long as possible is a lifestyle modification that should be lifelong.

What to Eat

Compliant Foods
- Lower-Protein Foods
- Chili con carne
- Beef stew
- Egg substitutes
- Tofu
- Imitation crabmeat
- Monounsaturated Fats
- Corn oil
- Safflower oil
- Olive oil
- Peanut oil
- Canola oil
- Low-Sodium Foods
- Salt-free herb seasonings
- Low-sodium canned foods
- Fresh, cooked meat
- Plain rice without sauce
- Plain noodles without sauce
- Fresh vegetables without sauce

- Frozen vegetables without sauce
- Homemade soup with fresh ingredients
- Reduced-sodium tomato sauce
- Unsalted pretzels
- Unsalted popcorn

Noncompliant Foods

- Higher-Protein Foods
- Ground beef
- Halibut
- Shrimp
- Salmon
- Tuna
- Chicken breast
- Roasted chicken
- Saturated fats
- Red meat
- Poultry
- Whole milk
- Butter
- Lard
- Trans-fatty acids
- Commercially baked goods
- French fries
- Doughnuts
- Hydrogenated vegetable oils

- Margarine
- Shortening
- High-Sodium Foods
- Salt
- Regular canned vegetables
- Hotdogs and canned meat
- Packaged rice with sauce
- Packaged noodles with sauce
- Frozen vegetables with sauce
- Frozen prepared meals
- Canned soup
- Regular tomato sauce
- Snack foods

Other Foods to Consider

Other types of foods that you may want to add to your diet are those with low potassium or phosphorus. You may also want to avoid foods and beverages with high levels of these minerals. However, with good kidney function, avoiding foods with these minerals may not always be necessary. Your healthcare provider may recommend specific restrictions if needed.

What to Include
Foods Lower in Potassium

- Apples, peaches
- Carrots, green beans
- White bread and pasta
- White rice
- Rice milk (not enriched)
- Cooked rice and wheat cereals, grits
- Apple, grape, or cranberry juice

Foods Lower in Phosphorous
- Fresh fruits and vegetables
- Breads, pasta, rice
- Rice milk (not enriched)
- Corn and rice cereals
- Light-colored sodas, such as lemon-lime or homemade iced tea

What to Avoid

Foods Higher in Potassium
- Oranges, bananas, and orange juice
- Potatoes, tomatoes
- Brown and wild rice
- Bran cereals
- Dairy foods
- Whole-wheat bread and pasta
- Beans and nuts

Foods Higher in Phosphorous

- Meat, poultry, fish
- Bran cereals and oatmeal
- Dairy foods
- Beans, lentils, nuts
- Dark-colored sodas, fruit punch, some bottled or canned iced teas that have added phosphorus

DASH diet

Studies in high blood pressure patients without PKD have shown that the so-called DASH diet (Dietary Approach to Stopping Hypertension), which consists of lots of fruits and vegetables combined with low-fat dairy, may lower blood pressure. A diet based on these guidelines could also seem appropriate for you. Look in the resources section at the back of the book for web resources on the DASH diet. Talk to your doctor before significantly altering your diet.

Example of a Renal Diet 1

Breakfast: One serving of egg substitute, scrambled with fresh chopped onion and red and green bell

peppers. Pair with one slice of white toast with one or two teaspoons of cream cheese and a small bowl (about a ½ cup) of fresh strawberries.
Snack: One apple, medium in size.
Lunch: Cabbage rolls-use two or three large, crisp, cabbage leaves to roll up shredded baked chicken, chopped apple, onions, a little bit of mayonnaise, and a sprinkle of honey mustard vinaigrette (made by whisking together apple cider vinegar, yellow mustard, and honey). Serve with a serving of unsalted pretzels.
Snack: One serving of baby carrots, with homemade, low sodium hummus or ranch dressing.
Dinner: Low sodium turkey and vegetable chili, topped with a small dollop of low fat sour cream. Serve with five unsalted crackers.
Dessert: Small slice of angel food cake with fresh strawberries and low fat, non-dairy whipped cream

Example of a renal diet 2

Breakfast: One English muffin with one teaspoon of cream cheese and one teaspoon of sugar free fruit preserve. Side with ½ cup of yellow grits and a small bowl of mixed berries.
Snack: One small bunch of grapes.

Lunch: ½ cup Cauliflower and ¼ cup chopped red bell pepper, sautéed in 1 tbsp olive oil with garlic and chopped onion. Toss with ½ cup of cooked noodles. Sprinkle with grated Parmesan cheese.

Snack: ½ cup peach slices with ¼ cup cottage cheese.

Dinner: Two chicken tacos, topped with a small amount of natural shredded cheese, chopped onions, and shredded cabbage. Serve with ½ cup of rice, seasoned with cilantro and lime juice.

Dessert: One medium apple, sliced and baked with cinnamon.

Chapter 4

Natural remedies and complications

Natural remedies can complement conventional medical treatments for poly-cystic kidney disease (PKD) and may help manage symptoms, support kidney function, and improve overall well-being. While natural remedies should not replace medical care or prescribed treatments, they can be used as part of a holistic approach to kidney health.

Commonly used herbs in PDK

Always consult your Clinical/Medical Herbalist before starting new herbs, do not self-dose. This is not a complete herbal list. If you take pharmaceuticals, please consult your physician.

Parsley Piert (Aphanes arvensis)
This herb is considered to be specific for the urinary tract as a whole and is cooling, demulcent, and a gentle diuretic. It is specific for renal calculi of

various types and for general kidney and bladder problems. Also specific in issues when edema is caused by renal dysfunction. There are no known contraindications with current medications, however, due to lack of research it is best to avoid in pregnancy and lactation. Additionally, it is best taken as an infusion (tea).

Couch Grass (Elymus repens)
This traditional herb is one that I would consider to be a specific when pairing with other herbs for PKD. It is considered to be anti-inflammatory, demulcent, anti-bacterial and anti-microbial which can help against the possibility of secondary infection within the kidney. It is also considered tonic to the urinary tract which means it can potentially assist with the balance of proper function.

Nettle Seed (Urtica dioica)
One of my first cases post graduation was a client in hospital with kidney failure who was not responding to conventional drugs. By request of the client, I was allowed to enter the hospital in order to give him herbs (this is not in any way the norm, and I think at the time there was a very frustrated physician) The client was given high doses of nettle seed, and though he did not make a full recovery, he was later

stable enough to be discharged (due to lack of research, and this being a singular case, I cannot state with full certainty that this herb was the singular cause since other herbs, and pharmaceuticals were involved). Nettle seed is a powerful herbal ally when it comes to kidney function and bringing down inflammation in the kidney. It is considered to be a highly respected kidney trophorestorative herbs. In some initial clinical studies it has been shown to slow down renal failure, and increase kidney glomerular function and lowered serum creatine levels. For a bit more commentary on Nettle Seed, please see the article attached here.

Marshmallow (Althea officinalis)
This is an herb that I would consider as a specific in any disorders of inflammation in the mucosal membrane of the body. From the gastrointestinal tract, to the full function of the urinary system, marshmallow is excellent as a soothing anti-inflammatory. It is also considered to be protective of the mucosal lining due to its mucilagenous properties, and is a key anti-irritant. It is a specific for inflammation within the kidney and bladder, and any sort of chronic irritation to the system as a whole.

Again, this is by no means an inclusive list, as depending on the individual case I would no doubt use variety of far more powerful herbs. However, in my opinion these are good general usage herbs that can be paired with specifics for an individual formulation.

Acupuncture
A component of traditional Chinese medicine, involves the insertion of thin needles into specific points on the body to promote balance and alleviate symptoms. Some individuals with PKD may find acupuncture helpful for managing pain, reducing stress, and improving overall well-being.

Complications

Complications associated with polycystic kidney disease include:

High blood pressure
Elevated blood pressure is a common complication of polycystic kidney disease. Untreated, high blood pressure can cause further damage to your kidneys and increase your risk of heart disease and strokes.

Managing HBP

Managing high blood pressure in polycystic kidney disease (PKD) is crucial to slow the progression of kidney damage and reduce the risk of complications like cardiovascular disease. Here are some strategies for managing high blood pressure in PKD:

1. Healthy Diet: Adopting a healthy diet can help control blood pressure. Focus on eating plenty of fruits, vegetables, whole grains, and lean proteins. Limit sodium intake, as excessive sodium can raise blood pressure. Aim for less than 2,300 milligrams of sodium per day, or even less if your doctor recommends it.

2. Exercise Regularly: Regular physical activity can help lower blood pressure and improve overall health. Aim for at least 150 minutes of moderate-intensity exercise, such as brisk walking, each week. Always consult with your healthcare provider before starting any new exercise regimen.

3. Maintain a Healthy Weight: Being overweight or obese can increase blood pressure. Losing weight through a combination of healthy eating and regular

exercise can help lower blood pressure and improve kidney function.

4. Limit Alcohol and Caffeine: Alcohol and caffeine can raise blood pressure, so it's best to consume them in moderation. Limit alcohol intake to no more than one drink per day for women and two drinks per day for men. Be mindful of caffeinated beverages like coffee, tea, and soda.

5. Quit Smoking: Smoking can raise blood pressure and further damage your kidneys. If you smoke, quitting is one of the best things you can do for your overall health.

6. Manage Stress: Chronic stress can contribute to high blood pressure. Practice stress-reducing techniques such as deep breathing, meditation, yoga, or spending time on hobbies you enjoy.

7. Monitor Blood Pressure Regularly: Keep track of your blood pressure at home using a home blood pressure monitor. This can help you and your doctor monitor how well your treatment plan is working and make adjustments as needed.

Remember, managing high blood pressure in PKD requires a comprehensive approach involving medication, lifestyle changes, and regular medical care. Always consult with your healthcare provider before making any significant changes to your treatment plan.

Loss of kidney function
Progressive loss of kidney function is one of the most serious complications of polycystic kidney disease. Nearly half of those with the disease have kidney failure by age 60.

PKD can interfere with the ability of your kidneys to keep wastes from building to toxic levels, a condition called uremia. As the disease worsens, end-stage kidney (renal) disease may result, necessitating ongoing kidney dialysis or a transplant to prolong your life.

Managing Loss of Kidney Function
Loss of kidney function, especially in conditions like polycystic kidney disease (PKD), can have significant implications for your health. Here's some information about the potential consequences and how to manage them:

1. Progression of Kidney Disease: In PKD, cysts grow in the kidneys, gradually replacing healthy tissue and impairing kidney function. As kidney function declines, waste products and excess fluid can build up in the body, leading to symptoms such as fatigue, swelling, nausea, and difficulty concentrating.

2. High Blood Pressure: Chronic kidney disease (CKD), including PKD, often leads to high blood pressure (hypertension) due to the kidneys' role in regulating blood pressure. High blood pressure, in turn, can further damage the kidneys, creating a vicious cycle.

3. Fluid and Electrolyte Imbalance: As kidney function declines, the kidneys may struggle to maintain the body's balance of fluids and electrolytes (such as sodium, potassium, and calcium). This can lead to complications like edema (swelling), electrolyte imbalances, and acid-base disturbances.

4. Anemia: Healthy kidneys produce a hormone called erythropoietin, which stimulates the production of red blood cells. As kidney function decreases, erythropoietin production declines,

leading to anemia (low red blood cell count) and its associated symptoms, such as fatigue and weakness.

5. Bone and Mineral Disorders: The kidneys play a crucial role in maintaining bone health by regulating calcium and phosphorus levels. As kidney function declines, imbalances in these minerals can occur, leading to bone disorders like osteoporosis and renal osteodystrophy.

6. Cardiovascular Disease: CKD is a significant risk factor for cardiovascular disease, including heart attacks, strokes, and peripheral artery disease. High blood pressure, fluid retention, and metabolic changes associated with kidney disease contribute to this increased risk.

7. End-stage Renal Disease (ESRD): In advanced stages of kidney disease, when kidney function is severely impaired, a condition known as end-stage renal disease develops. At this stage, the kidneys can no longer function well enough to sustain life without dialysis or kidney transplantation.

Managing the loss of kidney function in PKD involves a combination of medical treatments, lifestyle modifications, and regular monitoring. This may include:

- Dietary Changes: Following a kidney-friendly diet that is low in sodium, potassium, and phosphorus can help reduce the strain on the kidneys and manage complications like high blood pressure and electrolyte imbalances.

- Fluid Restriction: In later stages of kidney disease, fluid intake may need to be restricted to prevent fluid overload and swelling.

- Regular Monitoring: Regular blood tests, urine tests, and blood pressure checks are essential for monitoring kidney function and managing complications.

- Lifestyle Modifications: Quitting smoking, maintaining a healthy weight, exercising regularly, and managing stress can help slow the progression of kidney disease and reduce the risk of complications.

- Dialysis or Kidney Transplant: In cases of ESRD, dialysis or kidney transplantation may be necessary to sustain life. These treatments replace the lost kidney function and can significantly improve quality of life and long-term outcomes.

Managing the loss of kidney function in PKD requires a multidisciplinary approach involving nephrologists, dietitians, and other healthcare professionals. It's essential to work closely with your healthcare team to develop a personalized treatment plan that addresses your specific needs and concerns.

Chronic pain

Pain is a common symptom for people with polycystic kidney disease. It often occurs in your side or back. The pain can also be associated with a urinary tract infection, a kidney stone or a malignancy.

Growth of cysts in the liver

The likelihood of developing liver cysts for someone with poly-cystic kidney disease increases with age. While both men and women develop cysts, women often develop larger cysts. Female hormones and multiple pregnancies might contribute to liver cyst development.

Managing Growth of Cysts in the Liver

In poly-cystic liver disease (PLD), cysts develop in the liver, leading to enlargement and potential complications. Managing the growth of cysts in the liver is essential for controlling symptoms and preventing complications. Here's how it can be addressed:

1. Regular Monitoring: People with PLD should undergo regular imaging tests, such as ultrasounds or MRIs, to monitor the size and number of liver cysts. This helps track disease progression and guide treatment decisions.

2. Symptom Management: Treatment may focus on managing symptoms associated with enlarged liver cysts, such as abdominal pain, fullness, or discomfort. Over-the-counter pain relievers or prescription medications may be recommended to alleviate symptoms.

3. Surgery: In some cases, surgery may be necessary to drain large cysts or remove part of the liver (hepatic resection) to relieve symptoms or prevent complications. However, surgery carries risks and is typically reserved for individuals with severe symptoms or complications.

5. Lifestyle Modifications: Making lifestyle changes, such as maintaining a healthy weight, avoiding alcohol, and eating a balanced diet low in sodium and fat, may help manage symptoms and support overall liver health.

6. Management of Complications: PLD can lead to complications such as infection, rupture of cysts, or compression of nearby organs. Prompt medical attention is necessary if complications occur.

7. Genetic Counseling: PLD can be inherited, so individuals with a family history of the disease may benefit from genetic counseling to understand their risk and make informed decisions about family planning.

It's important for individuals with PLD to work closely with a healthcare provider experienced in managing liver diseases. Treatment decisions should be tailored to each person's specific symptoms, disease severity, and overall health. Regular follow-up appointments and monitoring are crucial to ensure that treatment remains effective and complications are promptly addressed.

Development of an aneurysm in the brain

A balloon-like bulge in a blood vessel (aneurysm) in your brain can cause bleeding (hemorrhage) if it ruptures. People with poly-cystic kidney disease have a higher risk of aneurysms. People with a family history of aneurysms seem to be at highest risk. Ask your doctor if screening is needed in your case. If screening reveals that you don't have an aneurysm, your doctor may recommend repeating the screening exam in a few years or after several years as a follow-up. The timing of repeat screening depends on your risk.

Pregnancy complications

Pregnancy is successful for most women with poly-cystic kidney disease. In some cases, however, women may develop a life-threatening disorder called pre-eclampsia. Those most at risk have high blood pressure or a decline in kidney function before they become pregnant.

Heart valve abnormalities

As many as 1 in 4 adults with poly-cystic kidney disease develops mitral valve prolapse. When this happens, the heart valve no longer closes properly, which allows blood to leak backward.

Colon problems
Weaknesses and pouches or sacs in the wall of the colon (diverticulosis) may develop in people with poly-cystic kidney disease.

Chapter 5

Caregiver and coping with PKD

Caring for someone with poly-cystic kidney disease (PKD) presents unique challenges that extend beyond managing the physical aspects of the condition. Caregivers play a vital role in providing emotional support, assistance with daily activities, and navigating the complexities of healthcare. However, the care giving journey can be emotionally taxing and physically demanding, requiring caregivers to develop coping strategies and seek support to maintain their well-being.

Caregivers of individuals with PKD often find themselves juggling multiple responsibilities, from managing medication regimens to accompanying their loved ones to medical appointments. The unpredictability of the disease and the uncertainty surrounding its progression can add to the stress and anxiety experienced by caregivers. Additionally, witnessing the physical and emotional toll that PKD takes on their loved ones can be emotionally challenging for caregivers, leading to feelings of helplessness, frustration, and sadness.

In the midst of care giving responsibilities, it's essential for caregivers to prioritize their own well-being and practice self-care. This may involve setting boundaries, taking breaks when needed, and seeking support from family, friends, or support groups. Connecting with other caregivers who understand the challenges firsthand can provide a sense of validation, comfort, and encouragement. Online forums, support groups, and local organizations dedicated to PKD can be valuable resources for caregivers seeking community and peer support.

Coping with the demands of care giving also requires caregivers to cultivate resilience and develop effective coping strategies. Engaging in activities that promote relaxation, such as meditation, yoga, or spending time in nature, can help reduce stress and restore a sense of balance. Prioritizing self-care activities, such as regular exercise, healthy eating, and adequate sleep, is essential for maintaining physical and emotional well-being.

Effective communication is key to navigating the caregiver role and fostering a supportive relationship with the individual with PKD. Openly discussing concerns, needs, and preferences can help caregivers and their loved ones feel heard, understood, and supported. Establishing clear channels of communication with healthcare providers is also important for staying informed about treatment options, managing symptoms, and addressing any concerns or questions that may arise.

Ultimately, care-giving for someone with PKD is a journey that requires compassion, resilience, and adaptability. By practicing self-care, seeking support, and communicating openly, caregivers can navigate the challenges of care-giving while providing compassionate care and support for their loved ones with PKD.

Additional Resources

1. National Kidney Foundation (NKF): A leading organization dedicated to the awareness, prevention, and treatment of kidney disease. NKF provides educational resources, support services, and advocacy efforts for individuals affected by kidney disease and their families. Website: kidney.org

2. PKD Foundation: A nonprofit organization focused on advancing research, advocacy, and support for individuals and families affected by polycystic kidney disease (PKD). The PKD Foundation offers educational materials, support groups, fundraising events, and research funding opportunities. Website: pkdcure.org

3. American Association of Kidney Patients (AAKP): A patient-led organization dedicated to improving the lives of kidney patients through education, advocacy, and support. AAKP provides resources, publications, online communities, and advocacy initiatives for kidney patients and their caregivers. Website: aakp.org

4. Renal Support Network (RSN): A nonprofit organization that provides support, education, and empowerment to individuals affected by kidney disease. RSN offers peer support, educational materials, patient advocacy resources, and wellness programs for kidney patients and their families. Website: rsnhope.org

5. Kidney Community Emergency Response (KCER) Program: A federal initiative aimed at improving emergency preparedness and response for individuals with kidney disease. KCER provides resources, guidance, and educational materials on emergency planning, dialysis care during emergencies, and disaster recovery for kidney patients and providers. Website: kcercoalition.com

6. American Kidney Fund (AKF): A nonprofit organization dedicated to providing financial assistance, education, and support services to kidney patients in need. AKF offers programs to help kidney patients afford health insurance premiums, medications, transportation to dialysis, and other essential services. Website: kidneyfund.org

7. Dialysis Facility Compare: An online tool provided by the Centers for Medicare & Medicaid Services (CMS) that allows users to compare the quality of dialysis facilities based on various measures, including patient outcomes, infection rates, and patient satisfaction scores. Website: medicare.gov/dialysisfacilitycompare

8. ClinicalTrials.gov: A database of privately and publicly funded clinical studies conducted around the world. Individuals with kidney disease may find information about ongoing clinical trials investigating new treatments, interventions, and diagnostic tools for kidney disease and related conditions. Website: clinicaltrials.gov

9. Renal friendly cookbooks: There are lots of renal friendly cookbooks that would be very helpful to you. A few I recommend are:
Renal Harmony by Chris Kola
Renal Diet cookbook by Ella S. Woolery
Renal diet cookbook for beginners by Rose Foster

www.ingramcontent.com/pod-product-compliance
Lightning Source LLC
Chambersburg PA
CBHW050100230526
45470CB00004B/1613